# HOW TO STOP COUGHING

## A Complete Guide To
## Acute & Chronic Coughs
## Over 100 Proven Methods

Johnson Wu

**Loons Press**

FIRST EDITION

This publication is intended to provide educational information for the reader on the covered subjects. It is not intended to take the place of personalized medical counseling, diagnosis, and treatment from a trained healthcare professional.

Library and Archives Canada Cataloguing in Publication

ISBN 978-1-7387821-6-1 (Hardcover)
ISBN 978-1-7387821-8-5 (Paperback)
ISBN 978-1-7387821-4-7 (eBook)
ISBN 978-1-7387821-7-8 (Audiobook)

Printed and bound in USA
Published by Loons Press

*For Wei*

# TABLE OF CONTENT

# *PREFACE*

C oughing is a ubiquitous and often irritating symptom that can result from a broad range of causes, ranging from minor inconvenience to chronic and persistent issues. This symptom has become even more prevalent due to the rise of environmental irritants such as air pollution and allergens. Coughing can be a sign of a significant health problem and can have a major impact on daily life, whether it is an acute or chronic issue. People are constantly searching for effective methods to alleviate coughing and find relief from this discomforting symptom.

This book is written to provide practical solutions for coughing problems. It offers a comprehensive overview of the causes of coughing, including common colds and flu, as well as more severe conditions like asthma and bronchitis, and provides a wide range of evidence-based and effective strategies, with over 100 proven ways to stop coughing.

The focus of the book is on over 100 proven methods to alleviate coughing, including over-the-counter cough medicines, natural remedies such as honey and lemon, and lifestyle changes like dietary modifications and avoiding triggers like second-hand smoke. Alternative therapies, including acupuncture, herbal remedies, homeopathy, and traditional Chinese medicine, are also covered. From conventional treatments to natural remedies, the book presents a comprehensive list of solutions for managing coughing effectively. The book also offers practical tips for managing chronic coughs, such as staying hydrated and maintaining good respiratory hygiene, as well as information on when to seek medical attention and what to expect from a healthcare provider.

The author offers a balanced perspective on treatment, highlighting the pros and cons of both natural and conventional remedies, and providing clear explanations of the science behind various treatments, including their mechanisms of action, potential side effects, and when it's best to use each approach. In addition to information on how to stop coughing, the book also includes tips for preventing coughing, such as maintaining good respiratory health, reducing exposure to irritants, and improving overall immunity. The book also delves into the emotional impact that persistent coughing can have, including feelings of frustration, exhaustion, and isolation, and provides strategies for coping with these challenges. A comprehensive overview of the role of different healthcare professionals in the treatment of coughing, including therapists, alternative health practitioners, and physicians, is also included. This information is vital for anyone seeking the best possible care and treatment for their coughing symptoms.

In conclusion, this book is a valuable resource for anyone seeking a comprehensive and evidence-based guide to stopping coughing. Whether you are a healthcare professional, a patient, or someone who wants to learn more about coughing and related health issues, this book provides valuable information and practical strategies to help you achieve relief for coughing and improve your overall health and well-being.

# CHAPTER 1

## Introduction

## *The Pathophysiology of Coughing and Its Types*

C oughing refers to the forceful exhalation of air from the lungs, which serves to clear obstructions in the airway. Productive coughing is characterized by the expulsion of mucus or phlegm, whereas unproductive coughing, also known as dry coughing, does not result in the production of any substances.

Your lungs are a pair of spongy, air-filled organs located on either side of the chest (thorax). The trachea conducts inhaled air into the lungs through its tubular branches (bronchi). The bronchi then divide into smaller and smaller tubes called bronchioles, which eventually lead to tiny air sacs called alveoli. The alveoli are lined with very small blood vessels called capillaries.

The main function of the lungs is to exchange oxygen and carbon dioxide with the atmosphere, a process called gas exchange. When you inhale, air travels down the trachea and into the bronchi, which then branch off into smaller bronchioles. The bronchioles lead to the alveoli, which are surrounded by capillaries. Oxygen from the inhaled air passes through the alveoli walls and into the capillaries, where it is picked up by red blood cells and transported to the body's cells. At the same time, carbon dioxide, a waste product of cellular metabolism, passes from the body's cells into the capillaries and is exhaled out of the body.

The muscles of the chest and diaphragm control breathing. The diaphragm, a large muscle located under the lungs, contracts and flattens during inspiration (inhaling), expanding the chest cavity and drawing air into the lungs. The reverse happens during expiration (exhaling), when the diaphragm relaxes and the chest muscles contract, pushing air out of the lungs.

As you inhale, air passes through your nose or mouth, down your windpipe, and into your lungs. As the air passes through the windpipe and into the smaller airways (called bronchi), tiny hair-like structures called cilia move back and forth in coordinated waves, helping to sweep mucus and other substances out of the lungs. Coughing helps to clear the airways of mucus and other substances that can cause congestion or block the flow of air.

When sensors in the respiratory tract detect irritants or substances that need to be cleared from the airways. These sensors send a signal to the cough center in the brain, which initiates the cough reflex. Your brain cough center sends a signal to the respiratory muscles to contract. The main muscle involved in coughing is the diaphragm, which is a large muscle located between the chest and abdomen. Your diaphragm contracts and pushes down, increasing the pressure in the chest. At the same time, the muscles between the ribs contract, further increasing the pressure in the chest. The larynx (voice box) closes, and the epiglottis (a small, flap-like structure at the base of the tongue) covers the trachea (windpipe). This prevents food and liquids from entering the airways. As the pressure in the chest increases, the airways in the lungs expand and the air in the lungs is forced out rapidly. The rapid expulsion of air creates a loud, distinctive sound. The larynx and epiglottis open, and the air rushing out of the lungs creates a loud, distinctive sound. The air rushing out of your lungs helps to clear the airways of mucus and other substances that can cause congestion or block the flow of air.

Coughing is a natural reflex action that plays a crucial role in maintaining the health of the respiratory system. It is a protective mechanism that helps to clear the throat and airways of irritants or excess mucus, which can impede breathing and lead to infection. The reflex is triggered when something irritates the throat or airways, causing nerves to send a signal to the brain. The brain then signals the muscles in the chest and abdomen to forcefully push air out of the lungs to remove the irritant.

An occasional cough is normal. If a cough persists for several weeks or one that brings up discolored or bloody mucus may indicate an underlying condition that requires medical attention. It is a common symptom of many respiratory conditions and can be caused by a variety of factors, including infections (such as the common cold, flu, or bronchitis), allergies, irritants (such as cigarette smoke), and certain medical conditions (such as asthma or acid reflux).

However, when coughing becomes chronic or persistent, it can be a symptom of an underlying health problem. Chronic coughing can be caused by a wide range of factors, including respiratory conditions and heart disease, and certain medications. It can also be caused by environmental factors such as pollution, and allergens. Prolonged, vigorous coughing can also cause additional problems such as fatigue, dizziness, headaches, and even incontinence. Moreover, it can be a symptom of various underlying conditions such as pneumonia, even lung cancer.

The importance of finding a solution to coughing cannot be overstated. Chronic coughing can lead to a few negative consequences, including difficulty sleeping, chest pain, and even rib fractures. It can also be a significant source of stress and anxiety and can negatively impact one's quality of life. In some cases, chronic coughing can be a sign of a more serious underlying condition and seeking medical attention is important.

This book aims to provide a comprehensive guide to understanding the causes of coughing and the various methods that can be used to find relief. From lifestyle changes and home remedies to over-the-counter medications and medical treatments, readers will find a wide range of strategies for managing and treating their coughing.

Treatment for coughing depends on the underlying cause. For acute coughs caused by viral infections, over-the-counter medications such as cough syrups, lozenges, and decongestants can help relieve symptoms. In some cases, a healthcare professional may prescribe antibiotics or other medications to help treat the underlying condition causing the cough. For chronic coughs or coughs caused by underlying conditions, treatment may involve medications such as bronchodilators, corticosteroids, or proton pump inhibitors (PPIs) to address the underlying condition. In some cases, antibiotics may be prescribed if a bacterial infection is suspected.

In addition to medication, there are also lifestyle changes that can help alleviate coughing. These include quitting smoking, avoiding known irritants, using a humidifier to keep the air moist, and drinking plenty of fluids to help thin mucus. It's also important to maintain good overall health by eating a balanced diet, getting regular exercise, and getting enough sleep. The book also includes information on alternative therapies such as acupuncture, aromatherapy, and traditional Chinese medicine, as well as Mind-body therapies. The book will also discuss how to manage coughing associated with specific conditions such as asthma and allergies, coughing in children, even ancient medicine for coughing.

It's important to note that a cough can be a symptom of a more serious condition, such as lung cancer, tuberculosis, or lung embolism, and should be evaluated by a healthcare professional if it persists for more than a few weeks or is accompanied by other symptoms such as chest pain, shortness of breath, or a fever.

Always consult a qualified healthcare professional for prompt diagnosis and formal treatment. Please be reasonable and rational to consider any proper natural remedies to treat your coughing for a good therapeutic effect.

In summary, whether you are dealing with a minor cough or a more serious condition, this book will provide you with the information and tools you need to find relief. By understanding the causes of coughing and the available treatment options, readers will be better equipped to manage their symptoms and improve their quality of life.

Coughing can vary in intensity, duration, and frequency. It can be classified into different types depending on the underlying cause.

- **Acute cough** typically lasts less than three weeks and are often caused by a common cold, flu, or other respiratory infections. These types of coughs are usually accompanied by other symptoms such as a runny nose, sore throat, and fever.

- **Chronic cough (Persistent cough)** lasts longer than eight weeks and is often caused by underlying medical conditions such as asthma, chronic obstructive pulmonary disease (COPD), and gastroesophageal reflux disease (GERD). These types of coughs are usually accompanied by other symptoms such as difficulty breathing, chest pain, and a chronic productive cough. A chronic cough can have a significant impact on a person's quality of life and can lead to other complications such as chest pain, difficulty sleeping, and even weight loss.

- **Dry cough**: A dry cough is one that does not produce any phlegm or mucus. It is often caused by viral infections, such as the common cold, and can also be caused by environmental irritants, such as cigarette smoke or pollution.

- **Wet cough (Chesty cough)**: A wet cough, also known as a productive cough, is one that produces phlegm or mucus. It is often caused by bacterial infections, such as pneumonia, or by conditions such as asthma or bronchitis.

- **Nighttime cough**: A cough that occurs primarily at night can be caused by a variety of factors, including postnasal drip, acid reflux, or asthma.

- **Whooping cough**: A whooping cough, also known as pertussis, is a highly contagious bacterial infection that causes severe coughing spells that end in a "whooping" sound when the person inhales. This type of cough has been seen mostly in young children.

- **Barking coughing (croup),** is an inflammation of the larynx and trachea in children, associated with infection and causing breathing difficulties.

It's also important to understand that coughing can be caused by both underlying medical conditions or external factors such as pollution, dust, smoke, or certain chemicals. For example, exposure to second-hand smoke or air pollution can cause chronic coughing, especially in people with respiratory conditions such as asthma or chronic obstructive pulmonary disease (COPD).

# CHAPTER 2
## *The Causes of Coughing and Its Diagnosis*

C oughing is a common and complex physiological response that can be caused by a variety of factors. It is a protective mechanism that helps clear the airway of irritants and foreign substances. While coughing is a normal and healthy response to certain stimuli, it can also be a sign of an underlying health problem. Understanding the causes of coughing can help individuals identify the root cause of their symptoms and receive appropriate medical treatment.

One of the most common causes of coughing is respiratory viral infections such as the common cold, flu, bronchitis, or pneumonia. These infections cause inflammation in the airways, leading to increased mucus production and coughing. Additionally, respiratory infections can cause the airways to become narrow, making it difficult to breathe and leading to coughing fits. These types of coughs are usually accompanied by other symptoms such as a runny nose, sore throat, and fever.

Allergic reactions of Allergies and hay fever can also cause coughing, as the body tries to clear the airways of irritants such as pollen, dust, or pet dander, and other allergens. Allergic reactions can cause a range of symptoms, including sneezing, runny nose, and a persistent cough.

Asthma is another condition that can cause coughing, particularly in individuals with a history of respiratory problems. Asthma causes the airways to become inflamed, leading to narrowing and making it difficult to breathe, causing coughing and wheezing. Bronchitis is also a common cause of coughing, characterized by inflammation and swelling of the bronchial tubes, resulting in a persistent, persistent cough.

Cigarette smoking is another major cause of coughing, as the chemicals and irritants in cigarette smoke can damage the respiratory system. Smoking can irritate the airways, leading to inflammation and excessive mucus production, and cause coughing. Long-term exposure to second-hand smoke can also cause coughing and other respiratory symptoms. Additionally, exposure to air pollution and toxic substances in the workplace can also lead to coughing and other respiratory symptoms

Environmental irritants such as air pollution, dust, mold, and pet dander can also cause coughing. These irritants can cause inflammation in the airways, leading to coughing and other respiratory symptoms. In some individuals, exposure to these irritants can cause chronic coughing and even lead to the development of chronic obstructive pulmonary disease (COPD), including emphysema and chronic bronchitis, causes inflammation and narrowing of the airways, leading to coughing, wheezing, and shortness of breath

Gastroesophageal reflux disease (GERD), also known as acid reflux, can also cause coughing, as the contents of the stomach can flow back into the esophagus and irritate the airways, leading to coughing. This is particularly common in individuals who lie down after eating, as gravity can cause the contents of the stomach to flow back into the esophagus, particularly at night or after meals.

Coughing could also be from some causes like bronchiectasis, Tuberculosis, sarcoidosis, heart failure, or vocal cord dysfunction. Bronchiectasis is a condition in which the bronchial tubes become damaged and widen, causing chronic coughing, mucus production, and difficulty breathing. Tuberculosis (TB) is bacterial infection that primarily affects the lungs, causing persistent cough, chest pain, and difficulty breathing. Sarcoidosis is a disease characterized by the formation of tiny clusters of inflammatory cells in different parts of the body, including the lungs, leading to persistent cough, chest pain, and difficulty breathing. Heart failure is a condition in which the heart is not able to pump blood effectively, causing a buildup of fluids in the lungs, leading to a persistent cough, shortness of breath, and fatigue. Vocal cord dysfunction is a condition that causes the vocal cords to spasm and close, making it difficult to breathe and causing a persistent cough. In some cases, coughing can be a side effect of certain medications, including angiotensin-converting enzyme inhibitors (ACE inhibitors) and some types of pain medications. Persistent coughing can also be a symptom of certain medical conditions, such as lung cancer.

In conclusion, coughing is a common symptom that can be caused by a range of conditions, including the common cold, flu, asthma, bronchitis, allergic reactions, cigarette smoking, GERD, certain medications, and lower respiratory tract infections. If you are experiencing persistent coughing, it is important to seek medical attention to determine the underlying cause and receive appropriate treatment. By understanding the causes of coughing, individuals can take steps to prevent or manage the symptoms and maintain optimal respiratory health.

To diagnose the cause of a cough, a healthcare provider will typically take a patient's medical history, perform a physical examination, and order tests as needed.

- **Medical history:** The healthcare provider will ask the patient about their symptoms, including the duration and severity of the cough, as well as any other symptoms they may be experiencing, such as fever, shortness of breath, or chest pain. The healthcare provider will also ask about the patient's medical history, including any previous illnesses or conditions, and any medications they are currently taking.

- *Physical examination:* During the physical examination, the healthcare provider will listen to the patient's breathing with a stethoscope to help determine the location and severity of any abnormal sounds. They may also examine the patient's chest, looking for signs of infection or inflammation.

- *Chest X-ray:* This test creates images of the inside of the chest to help the healthcare provider look for signs of infection, inflammation, fluid in the lungs, or other abnormalities.

- *MRI or CT scan:* If the cough is accompanied by discolored or bloody mucus, MRI or CT scan may be performed to help to assess any additional symptoms or complications.

- *Spirometry:* This test measures how much air a person can exhale and how quickly they can exhale it. It can help diagnose conditions such as asthma or chronic obstructive pulmonary disease (COPD).

- *Pulmonary function test:* This test measures how well your lungs are working by measuring the amount of air you can inhale and exhale, and how quickly you can exhale. They may be used to diagnose conditions such as asthma or COPD.

- *Blood tests:* These tests can help your doctor determine if you have an infection or other underlying health condition that is causing your cough.

- *Bronchoscopy:* This test involves inserting a flexible tube with a light and camera into the airways through the nose or mouth. It allows the healthcare provider to see inside the airways and collect samples for further testing.

- *Allergy testing:* If your doctor thinks that your cough may be caused by an allergy, they may recommend allergy testing to determine the specific allergens that are causing your symptoms. Allergy testing could be skin or blood test.

- **Sputum culture:** This test involves collecting a sample of the mucus that is produced when you cough and testing it for bacteria or other microorganisms.

Although coughing is a common symptom, it can be caused by a number of serious conditions. If you have a persistent cough, it is important to consult with a healthcare provider, such as a pulmonologist. It is important to discuss your symptoms and concerns with your doctor so that they can recommend the most appropriate tests for your situation, to determine the underlying cause and appropriate treatment.

# CHAPTER 3

## *The Role of Immune System in Coughing*

To know the immune system's role in coughing, it is essential to understand the basic functions of the immune system and how it protects the body from pathogens and foreign substances. The immune system is a complex network of cells, tissues, and organs that work together to defend the body against harmful substances and infections. It is made up of two main branches, the innate and adaptive immune systems, which work together to protect the body.

The innate immune system is the first line of defense against infections and is activated immediately upon exposure to a pathogen or an irritant. It includes physical and chemical barriers, such as the skin, mucous membranes, and secretions, as well as immune cells, such as macrophages, neutrophils, and dendritic cells. These cells can engulf and destroy pathogens, as well as produce inflammation-causing substances, such as histamines, leukotrienes, and cytokines, to recruit and activate other immune cells.

The adaptive immune system is slower to respond to infections but is more specific and long-lasting. It includes immune cells, such as T cells and B cells, which can recognize and remember specific pathogens or substances. B cells produce antibodies, which can neutralize or eliminate pathogens. T cells can directly kill infected cells or stimulate other immune cells to do so. The adaptive immune system also includes the lymphatic system, which helps transport immune cells and substances throughout the body.

Coughing is a reflex that helps to clear the airways of mucus, irritants, and foreign particles. It is a protective mechanism that is triggered by various stimuli, such as exposure to an irritant, infection, or inflammation. Coughing is essential for maintaining proper respiratory function and can help to prevent infections from spreading throughout the body. The immune system plays a crucial role in this process by activating immune cells, releasing inflammation-causing substances, and producing antibodies. These antibodies help neutralize and eliminate pathogens, such as bacteria and viruses, that might cause a cough. The presence of antibodies in respiratory secretions, such as saliva and mucus, can indicate an ongoing immune response, which can contribute to coughing.

The immune system plays a crucial role in coughing, as it is responsible for detecting and eliminating foreign substances and pathogens from the body. When the body is exposed to a pathogen, such as a virus or bacterium, the immune system activates a response to eliminate it. This response involves activating immune cells and releasing substances that can cause inflammation, leading to symptoms such as coughing and sneezing. The immune system also creates antibodies that can be present in respiratory secretions and contribute to coughing. These substances work to protect the body by fighting the infection or removing the irritant but can also result in symptoms like coughing and congestion or leading to increased coughing. This increased coughing helps to remove the pathogens from the body and reduce the spread of the infection. The immune system and coughing work together to protect the body and maintain proper respiratory function.

In some cases, the immune system can overreact to respiratory infections or irritants, leading to chronic inflammation and persistent coughing, or increased coughing. This can happen in conditions such as asthma, COPD, and chronic bronchitis. On the other hand, a weakened or compromised immune system can make a person more susceptible to respiratory infections and persistent coughing. It is crucial for cough patients to work closely with their healthcare provider to determine the underlying cause and address it, including imbalances in the immune system.

Overall, the immune system plays a critical role in coughing, as it is responsible for detecting and eliminating foreign substances and pathogens from the body. The immune system and coughing work together to protect the body and maintain proper respiratory function. By exploring the relationship between the immune system and coughing, we can gain a deeper understanding of how the body protects itself, and how we can support and enhance its functions, and develop new treatments and therapies that can effectively target and improve respiratory health.

Exploring the relationship between the immune

system and coughing is critical for developing effective treatments and preventing respiratory illnesses. Here are some key elements to consider:

- **Inflammation:** Inflammation is a crucial part of the immune response. The immune system sends signals to surrounding tissues to initiate an inflammatory response when it detects an irritant in the respiratory system. This response helps clear the irritant and remove damaged tissues, and coughing can help remove the irritant and promote healing.

- **Mucus production:** Mucus production is a crucial aspect of the immune response. Mucus contains antibodies, antimicrobial peptides, and other immune substances that help trap and eliminate pathogens. Coughing helps remove mucus from the respiratory system and promotes proper respiratory function.

- **Immune cells:** The immune system has several types of immune cells that play a role in the response to irritants in the respiratory system. T-cells and B-cells coordinate the immune response and produce antibodies, while neutrophils, macrophages, and natural killer cells engulf and destroy pathogens. Dendritic cells present pathogens to T-cells, leading to an adaptive immune response.

- **Antibodies:** Antibodies are proteins produced

by the immune system in response to a specific pathogen. They help neutralize and remove the pathogen from the body, and coughing helps remove pathogens and antibodies from the respiratory system.

The respiratory system's defense mechanism, the immune system, plays a vital role in protecting the body from harmful substances and infections. For both patients suffering from a persistent cough and healthcare professionals, comprehending the immune system's involvement in coughing is of utmost importance in proper diagnosis and treatment of respiratory illnesses. When the body is exposed to pathogens, such as bacteria or viruses, the immune system activates a response to eliminate it, which can include coughing as a mechanism to remove the irritant from the respiratory system. In cases of infections, the immune system may produce cytokines and other substances causing inflammation in the airways and increased coughing to prevent the spread of the infection.

Treatment may involve the use of medications, such as antibiotics for respiratory infections, allergy medications, and inhalers for asthma and COPD, or lifestyle changes such as quitting smoking, avoiding irritants, managing stress, and improving diet and exercise to support the immune system. A personalized treatment plan, developed in collaboration with a healthcare provider, can address the specific needs of the patient and help them achieve better respiratory health.

In conclusion, the interplay between the immune system and coughing is a complex and crucial aspect of respiratory health. By understanding this relationship, cough patients can make informed decisions and take steps to improve their respiratory health, working closely with their healthcare provider to develop a tailored treatment plan.

# CHAPTER 4
## *Twenty-Seven Simple Home Remedies for Coughing*

Simple home remedies as a natural and cost-effective solution are a popular choice for treating coughing symptoms. One of the main reasons why home remedies are used for coughing is that they are often inexpensive and easily accessible. Many of the ingredients used in home remedies, such as honey, ginger, and lemon, can be found in most kitchens, making them a convenient and cost-effective option for those who are looking for a way to relieve their coughing symptoms.

Another reason why home remedies are used for coughing is that they are based on natural ingredients, which are safe for most people and have few side effects. For example, honey is a natural cough suppressant and has antibacterial properties that can help relieve sore throats, while ginger has anti-inflammatory properties that can help soothe irritated airways. By using natural remedies, people can avoid the harsh chemicals and artificial ingredients that are often found in over-the-counter medications.

Quick relief is another reason why people turn to home remedies for coughing. Drinking a warm beverage, such as tea with honey or lemon, can help soothe a sore throat. These remedies can provide quick relief from coughing symptoms, making them a popular choice for people who are looking for an effective and convenient solution. Meanwhile, home remedies can be used in addition to other treatments, such as medication, to help relieve coughing symptoms.

There are many reasons why home remedies are used for coughing, including:

1. *Simple:* Home remedies for coughing are simple to make and use:
2. *Cost-effective:* Home remedies are often inexpensive and easily accessible, making them a cost-effective solution for relieving coughing symptoms.
3. *Convenient:* Most home remedies can be made using ingredients that are commonly found in the kitchen, so they are convenient to use.
4. *Natural:* Home remedies are often based on natural ingredients, such as honey, ginger, and lemon, which are safe for most people and have few side effects.
5. *Quick relief:* Some home remedies, such as inhaling steam or drinking a warm beverage, can provide quick relief from coughing symptoms.
6. *Complementary treatment:* Home remedies can be used in addition to other treatments, such as medication, to help relieve coughing symptoms.

However, it's important to remember that while home remedies can provide relief, they may not be effective for everyone, and in some cases, a more serious underlying condition may be causing the cough. If your cough persists or worsens, a doctor should be consulted.

1.        *Honey:* Honey is a sweet substance produced by bees from the nectar of flowers. It contains a variety of nutrients, such as carbohydrates, enzymes, minerals, and vitamins, as well as antioxidants and other beneficial compounds. Honey has been used for centuries in traditional medicine to treat a variety of ailments, including coughs, due to its antimicrobial, anti-inflammatory, and expectorant properties. Honey can help relieve cough symptoms by coating the throat and suppressing cough reflexes, by reducing inflammation in the respiratory tract, and by eliminating or inhibiting the growth of respiratory pathogens. Honey can also boost the immune system by providing nutrients and antioxidants, and by stimulating the production of antibodies. Honey can be consumed on its own or added to teas, syrups, and other remedies to sweeten and enhance their flavor and effectiveness. It is important to note that honey should not be given to infants under 1 year of age due to the risk of botulism.

Mixing honey with warm water or tea can soothe a sore throat and help reduce coughing. Honey has natural anti-inflammatory and antimicrobial properties, and it can help to soothe a sore throat and suppress a cough.

Hot Honey Tea with lemon, or mint, or ginger, or cinnamon, or turmeric, or licorice root, or fennel, or anise, or clove, or cardamom, or black pepper, or cumin, or coriander, or lemon balm, or basil, or oregano, or thyme, whichever available or your favorite. Or simply just take a spoonful of honey before bedtime.

Honey can help reduce coughing, and hot tea can help soothe the throat, lemon and other natural herbs have antibacterial properties.

2. *Licorice:* Licorice is an herb that has been used for centuries to treat coughs and other respiratory conditions. Licorice is a demulcent, which means that it can help to soothe the lining of the respiratory tract and reduce inflammation. It has expectorant, antiviral, and anti-inflammatory properties that can help relieve cough symptoms and improve respiratory health. Licorice can be consumed in various forms, such as licorice tea, licorice supplements, or licorice tinctures. To use licorice for cough relief, you can try the following:

Licorice tea: Add a few dried licorice root slices to a cup of hot water. Let it steep for 5-10 minutes, then strain and drink. You can sweeten it with honey or another natural sweetener if desired. You can drink licorice tea 2-3 times a day as needed.

Licorice supplements: You can also take licorice supplements, such as licorice capsules or licorice extract, according to the instructions on the label. It is important to follow the recommended dosage and to consult with a healthcare professional before taking licorice supplements.

3. *Echinacea:* Echinacea is an herb that has been used for centuries to treat respiratory infections and boost the immune system. It has antiviral, immune-stimulating, and anti-inflammatory properties that can help reduce cough symptoms and improve respiratory health. Echinacea can be consumed in various forms, such as echinacea tea, echinacea supplements, or echinacea tinctures. To use echinacea for cough relief, you can try the following:

Echinacea tea: Add a few dried echinacea flowers or leaves to a cup of hot water. Let it steep for 5-10 minutes, then strain and drink. You can sweeten it with honey or another natural sweetener if desired. You can drink echinacea tea 2-3 times a day as needed.

Echinacea supplements: You can also take echinacea supplements, such as echinacea capsules or echinacea extract, according to the instructions on the label.

4.            *Garlic:* Garlic is a pungent herb that has been used for centuries in traditional medicine to treat a variety of ailments, including coughs. It contains a variety of nutrients, such as vitamins, minerals, and antioxidants, as well as beneficial compounds, such as allicin, that have antimicrobial, anti-inflammatory, and expectorant properties. Garlic can help relieve cough symptoms by reducing inflammation in the respiratory tract, by eliminating or inhibiting the growth of respiratory pathogens, and by breaking down and eliminating mucus. Garlic can also boost the immune system by providing nutrients, antioxidants, and other beneficial compounds, and by stimulating the production of antibodies.

Crush fresh garlic and mix it with honey to make a cough syrup. Garlic is a natural antibiotic and anti-inflammatory, which can help to reduce inflammation in the airways and soothe a cough. Try adding fresh garlic to your meals or taking a supplement.

5.            *Simple Herbal Tea:* Herbs such as ginger, thyme, and marshmallow root can help to soothe a sore throat, reduce inflammation, and relieve coughing. Drinking herbal teas that contain these herbs can help to provide relief.

i. Thyme: Thyme is an expectorant, which means that it can help to loosen mucus and make it easier to cough up.

ii. Marshmallow: Marshmallow is a demulcent that can help to soothe the throat and reduce irritation.

iii. Slippery elm: Slippery elm is a demulcent that can help to soothe the throat and reduce inflammation.

iv. Mullein: Mullein is an expectorant that can help to loosen mucus and make it easier to cough up.

6.        *Saltwater Gargle:* Saltwater gargle is a simple and effective home remedy that has been used for generations to relieve coughing symptoms. One of the main reasons why saltwater gargle is effective for coughing is that it helps soothe a sore throat. Sore throats can be caused by a variety of underlying conditions, including colds, flu, and sinus infections, and can make coughing symptoms worse. By gargling with warm salt water, people can relieve soreness and irritation in their throat, which can help

reduce coughing.

Saltwater gargle is also an effective remedy for coughing because it helps to clear nasal passages. When nasal passages are congested, it can be difficult to breathe and coughing can become more frequent. By gargling with salt water, people can help to clear mucus from their nasal passages and reduce coughing.

Another reason why saltwater gargle is used for coughing is that it is a natural and safe remedy. Unlike over-the-counter medications, which can have harsh chemicals and artificial ingredients, saltwater gargle is made from two simple and readily available ingredients: salt and water. This makes it a safe and natural choice for people who are looking for an affordable and effective way to relieve coughing symptoms.

Saltwater gargle is also a convenient remedy for coughing. It can be made quickly and easily at home, and can be used at any time of day. This makes it a popular choice for people who are looking for a quick and easy solution to relieve coughing symptoms. By using saltwater gargle, people can find relief from coughing symptoms in a safe and natural way, without having to rely on over-the-counter medications.

7.        *Chicken Soup:* Chicken soup has been used as a home remedy for centuries to relieve symptoms of coughing and colds. This simple, yet nourishing soup is believed to have medicinal properties that can help

soothe a sore throat, reduce inflammation, and boost the immune system.

One of the main reasons why chicken soup is effective for coughing is that it can help soothe a sore throat. A sore throat is a common symptom of colds, flu, and other respiratory infections, and can make coughing symptoms worse. By drinking warm chicken soup, people can relieve soreness and irritation in their throat, which can help reduce coughing.

Chicken soup is also believed to have anti-inflammatory properties that can help reduce inflammation in the body. Inflammation can contribute to coughing symptoms, particularly in cases of bronchitis or pneumonia. By consuming chicken soup, people can help reduce inflammation in their respiratory system and reduce coughing symptoms.

Another reason why chicken soup is used for coughing is that it is a nutritious and filling food. Chicken soup is a good source of protein, vitamins, and minerals, and can help to boost the immune system. This can be especially important for people with chronic or severe coughing symptoms, as a strong immune system can help fight off underlying infections.

Chicken soup is also a convenient and accessible remedy for coughing. It can be made easily at home or purchased pre-made from a grocery store. This makes it a popular choice for people who are looking for a quick and easy solution to relieve coughing symptoms.

8.        *Apple Cider Vinegar:* Apple cider vinegar is a versatile and commonly used ingredient in home remedies for various health issues, including coughing. This acidic liquid is believed to have anti-inflammatory and antimicrobial properties that can help relieve coughing symptoms and support overall health.

One of the main reasons why apple cider vinegar is effective for coughing is that it has antibacterial and antiviral properties. Many coughs and colds are caused by bacterial or viral infections, and apple cider vinegar can help to kill these pathogens and reduce symptoms. By consuming apple cider vinegar, people can help to eliminate underlying infections and reduce coughing symptoms. Apple cider vinegar is also believed to have anti-inflammatory properties that can help reduce inflammation in the body. Inflammation can contribute to coughing symptoms, particularly in cases of bronchitis or pneumonia. By consuming apple cider vinegar, people can help reduce inflammation in their respiratory system and reduce coughing symptoms.

Another reason why apple cider vinegar is used for coughing is that it is a natural and safe remedy. Unlike over-the-counter medications, which can have harsh chemicals and artificial ingredients, apple cider vinegar is made from natural ingredients and has a long history of safe use. This makes it a safe and natural choice for people who are looking for an affordable and effective way to relieve coughing symptoms.

To use apple cider vinegar as a remedy for coughing, it can be consumed directly or added to other remedies, such as tea or honey. One common method of using apple cider vinegar for coughing is to mix one or two tablespoons of apple cider vinegar with a glass of water and drink it three times a day. It is recommended to use raw, organic apple cider vinegar with the "mother" for best results. (The unfiltered and unrefined vinegar with cloudy and murky appearance is called apple cider vinegar with "mother". It is used for drinking purposes and has many health benefits due to the presence of beneficial bacteria, yeast and protein.)

Another popular method of using apple cider vinegar for coughing is to add it to a warm bath. This can help to relieve coughing symptoms by opening up airways and reducing inflammation. To do this, add one or two cups of apple cider vinegar to a warm bath and soak for 15-20 minutes.

It is important to note that apple cider vinegar is highly acidic and can cause irritation or damage to the skin or mucous membranes if not diluted properly. It is also recommended to avoid using undiluted apple cider vinegar internally for extended periods of time, as excessive consumption can lead to potential side effects such as decreased potassium levels and erosion of tooth enamel.

9.          *Radish Juice:* Radish juice is a popular home remedy for coughing and other respiratory issues. It is believed to have several health benefits that can help relieve coughing symptoms and support overall health.

Radishes are a rich source of vitamins and minerals, including vitamin C, folate, and potassium. These nutrients are essential for maintaining a healthy respiratory system and can help to reduce coughing symptoms. Vitamin C, in particular, is known for its ability to boost the immune system and fight off infections, making it a valuable ingredient in any home remedy for coughing.

Radish juice is also believed to have expectorant properties, which means it can help to loosen and remove mucus from the respiratory system. Mucus buildup can contribute to coughing symptoms, particularly in cases of bronchitis or pneumonia. By consuming radish juice, people can help to clear mucus from their respiratory system and reduce coughing symptoms.

To use radish juice as a remedy for coughing, it is recommended to consume one to two glasses of fresh radish juice per day. To make the juice, simply blend fresh radishes in a blender or juicer and strain the juice through a fine sieve. Radish juice can be consumed as is or mixed with other ingredients, such as honey or lemon juice, for added flavor and health benefits. Another best method is to steam big white radish (bai luo bo or Daikon) with rock sugar, drink the water and eat the radish, excellent result for coughing.

It is important to note that radish juice can be quite pungent and may not be suitable for everyone. Additionally, some people may experience digestive issues, such as bloating or gas, after consuming radish juice. If you experience any adverse reactions, it is recommended to discontinue use and seek medical advice if necessary.

10.    *Dandelion Leaves:* Dandelion leaves are commonly used in natural remedies for various health issues, including coughing. This plant is rich in vitamins and minerals, including vitamins A and C, as well as potassium and iron, which are beneficial for respiratory health.

One of the main reasons dandelion leaves are used for coughing is due to their ability to support liver function. The liver is responsible for eliminating toxins from the body, and when it is not functioning optimally, it can contribute to respiratory issues, including coughing. By supporting liver function, dandelion leaves can help to improve overall respiratory health and reduce coughing symptoms.

Dandelion leaves are also believed to have

anti-inflammatory properties, which can help to soothe the airways and reduce coughing. They contain compounds that can act as natural decongestants, reducing inflammation in the respiratory system and making it easier to breathe. This can help to relieve coughing and other symptoms associated with respiratory issues.

To use dandelion leaves for coughing, they can be consumed in several ways. Fresh dandelion leaves can be added to salads or blended into smoothies, or they can be dried and made into tea. To make dandelion tea, simply steep dried dandelion leaves in hot water for 10-15 minutes, then strain and drink as needed.

It is important to note that not all people are able to tolerate dandelion leaves and some may experience adverse reactions, such as digestive discomfort or skin irritation. Additionally, dandelion leaves can interact with certain medications, so it is important to consult with a healthcare professional before using them as a remedy for coughing or any other health issue.

11.     *Peppermint:* Peppermint is a well-known herb that has been used for centuries for its medicinal properties. It is commonly used to treat a variety of health issues, including coughing. Peppermint contains menthol, which is an organic compound that has a cooling and soothing effect on

the throat, making it a popular remedy for coughing. Peppermint can be a safe and effective remedy for controlling coughing by reducing irritation in the airways.

There are several ways to use peppermint for coughing. The most common method is to inhale the scent of peppermint oil, which is readily available in most health food stores. To use peppermint oil for coughing, simply add a few drops to a bowl of hot water and inhale the steam. This will help to open up the airways and relieve coughing.

Another popular way to use peppermint for coughing is to drink peppermint tea. Peppermint tea can be made by boiling fresh or dried peppermint leaves in water for several minutes. The menthol in the peppermint will help to soothe the throat and reduce coughing. Additionally, drinking warm liquids can also help to hydrate the throat, reducing dryness and irritation.

It's also possible to use peppermint oil for coughing by rubbing a few drops of the oil onto the chest and throat. The menthol in the oil will be absorbed through the skin and help to relieve coughing. This method is especially helpful for those who have trouble breathing through their nose.

It's important to note that peppermint should be used with caution, especially for those who are pregnant, breastfeeding, or have a history of heartburn. Peppermint can worsen heartburn and should be avoided by those with this condition.

12.        *Basil Leaves* Basil is a popular herb that has been used for centuries for its medicinal properties, including its ability to relieve coughing. Basil leaves contain compounds that have anti-inflammatory, antibacterial, and expectorant properties, making them an effective remedy for controlling coughing. Basil can help to relieve coughing by reducing inflammation and promoting the release of mucus, making it easier to breathe.

There are several ways to use basil leaves for coughing. The most common method is to make basil tea. To make basil tea, simply boil a handful of fresh basil leaves in water for several minutes. The tea can be sweetened with honey to taste and should be consumed several times a day to help relieve coughing.

Another way to use basil for coughing is to inhale the scent of basil essential oil. Basil essential oil can be added to a bowl of hot water and inhaled, or it can be added to a diffuser to be breathed in throughout the day. Inhaling the scent of basil can help to soothe the throat and reduce coughing.

It is also possible to use basil leaves for coughing by chewing on fresh basil leaves. Chewing on fresh basil leaves can help to stimulate the release of saliva, which can help to soothe the throat and reduce coughing. Additionally, basil leaves can be added to food and drinks, such as soups and smoothies, to help relieve coughing.

It is important to note that basil should be used with caution, especially for those who are pregnant, breastfeeding, or have a history of allergies. Overall, basil is a natural remedy that can be used to relieve coughing.

13.        *Turmeric*: Turmeric is a popular spice that is well known for its numerous health benefits, including its ability to relieve coughing. Turmeric contains curcumin, a compound with potent anti-inflammatory and antioxidant properties that makes it an effective remedy for controlling coughing. Turmeric can help to relieve coughing by reducing inflammation in the airways and promoting the release of mucus, making it easier to breathe.

There are several ways to use turmeric for coughing. The most common method is to drink turmeric milk, also known as "golden milk". To make turmeric milk, simply heat a glass of milk and add a teaspoon of turmeric powder, along with other spices such as cinnamon and black pepper, for enhanced flavor and health benefits. Drinking turmeric milk several times a day can help to soothe the throat and reduce coughing.

Another way to use turmeric for coughing

is to make a turmeric tea. To make turmeric tea, simply boil water with turmeric powder and other spices, such as ginger and black pepper, for several minutes. This tea can be consumed several times a day to help relieve coughing.

Turmeric can also be added to food and drinks, such as soups and smoothies, to help relieve coughing. Additionally, turmeric supplements can be taken in capsule form to help reduce coughing. However, it's important to consult with a healthcare provider before taking any supplements, as high doses of turmeric can interact with certain medications.

It is important to note that turmeric should be used with caution, especially for those who are pregnant, breastfeeding, or have a history of gallbladder issues.

14.        *Aloe vera:* Aloe vera is a succulent plant that has been used for centuries for its medicinal properties, including its ability to relieve coughing. Aloe vera contains compounds that have anti-inflammatory, antibacterial, and expectorant properties, making it an effective remedy for controlling coughing. Aloe vera can help to relieve coughing by reducing inflammation in the airways and promoting the release of mucus, making it easier to breathe.

There are several ways to use aloe vera for coughing. The most common method is to drink aloe vera juice. To make aloe vera juice, simply blend aloe vera gel with water and other ingredients, such as lemon juice and honey, for added flavor and health benefits. Drinking aloe vera juice several times a day can help to soothe the throat and reduce coughing.

Another way to use aloe vera for coughing is to apply aloe vera gel to the skin. Aloe vera gel can be applied directly to the chest, neck, and throat to help relieve coughing. This method works by reducing inflammation and promoting the release of mucus, making it easier to breathe.

Aloe vera can also be added to food and drinks, such as soups and smoothies, to help relieve coughing. Additionally, aloe vera supplements can be taken in capsule form to help reduce coughing. However, it's important to consult with a healthcare provider before taking any supplements, as high doses of aloe vera can interact with certain medications.

It is important to note that aloe vera should be used with caution, especially for those who are pregnant, breastfeeding, or have a history of gastrointestinal issues. Additionally, aloe vera can cause skin irritation in some individuals and should be used with care.

15.    *Clove:* Cloves are the aromatic flower buds of the clove tree that have been used for centuries for their medicinal properties, including their ability to relieve coughing. Cloves contain compounds that have antiseptic, anesthetic, and expectorant

properties, making them an effective remedy for controlling coughing. Cloves can help to relieve coughing by reducing inflammation in the airways, soothing the throat, and promoting the release of mucus, making it easier to breathe.

There are several ways to use cloves for coughing. The most common method is to make clove tea. To make clove tea, simply boil water with whole cloves and other ingredients, such as ginger and cinnamon, for several minutes. This tea can be consumed several times a day to help relieve coughing.

Another way to use cloves for coughing is to inhale clove oil. Clove oil can be added to boiling water and inhaled through the steam to help relieve coughing. This method works by reducing inflammation in the airways and soothing the throat.

Cloves can also be added to food and drinks, such as soups and smoothies, to help relieve coughing. Additionally, clove supplements can be taken in capsule form to help reduce coughing. However, it's important to consult with a healthcare provider before taking any supplements, as high doses of cloves can interact with certain medications.

It is important to note that cloves should be used with caution, especially for those who are pregnant, breastfeeding, or have a history of liver issues.

16.    *Fenugreek:*    Fenugreek,    also known as Trigonella foenum-graecum, is a commonly used herb in traditional medicine for various health issues, including coughing. One of the main reasons fenugreek is used for coughing is because it contains compounds that help reduce inflammation in the respiratory tract. This reduction in inflammation helps to relieve symptoms such as coughing, chest tightness, and difficulty breathing. Furthermore, fenugreek is also believed to possess expectorant properties, which help to loosen mucus and promote its removal from the respiratory tract. This can help to reduce coughing and prevent the buildup of harmful substances in the respiratory system.

In order to use fenugreek for coughing, it is important to understand the different forms in which the herb is available. Fenugreek can be found in the form of seeds, powder, capsules, and teas. The most commonly used forms for treating coughing are fenugreek tea and capsules.

To prepare fenugreek tea, simply boil one teaspoon of fenugreek seeds in a cup of water for about 10 minutes. Strain the mixture and drink the tea three times a day to help relieve coughing. Fenugreek capsules can be taken as directed by the manufacturer.

It is important to note that fenugreek should

not be used as a substitute for medical treatment for persistent or severe coughing. If your cough persists for more than a week, it is recommended that you seek medical attention.

> 17. ***Cardamom:*** Cardamom, scientifically known as Elettaria cardamomum, is a commonly used spice in traditional medicine for various health issues, including coughing. One of the main reasons cardamom is used for coughing is because it contains compounds that help reduce inflammation in the respiratory tract. This reduction in inflammation helps to relieve symptoms such as coughing, chest tightness, and difficulty breathing. Furthermore, cardamom is also believed to possess expectorant properties, which help to loosen mucus and promote its removal from the respiratory tract. This can help to reduce coughing and prevent the buildup of harmful substances in the respiratory system. Additionally, cardamom's antispasmodic properties can help to relieve chest tightness, which can often accompany coughing.

In order to use cardamom for coughing, it is important to understand the different forms in which the spice is available. Cardamom can be found in the form of seeds, powder, and oil. The most commonly used forms for treating coughing are cardamom tea and oil.

To prepare cardamom tea, simply boil a few crushed cardamom seeds in a cup of water for about 10 minutes. Strain the mixture and add honey to taste. Drink the tea three times a day to help relieve coughing. Cardamom oil can be added to hot water and inhaled to help relieve symptoms.

It is important to note that cardamom should not be used as a substitute for medical treatment for persistent or severe coughing. If your cough persists for more than a week, it is recommended that you seek medical attention. Additionally, individuals with certain medical conditions, such as heart problems or ulcers, should consult with their healthcare provider before using cardamom.

18. *Coriander*: Coriander, also known as cilantro or Chinese parsley, is a commonly used herb in traditional medicine for various health issues, including coughing. The main reason coriander is used for coughing is because it contains compounds that help reduce inflammation in the respiratory tract. This reduction in inflammation helps to relieve symptoms such as coughing, chest tightness, and difficulty breathing. Furthermore, coriander is also believed to possess expectorant properties, which help to loosen mucus and promote its removal from the respiratory tract.

This can help to reduce coughing and prevent the buildup of harmful substances in the respiratory system. Additionally, coriander's antispasmodic properties can help to relieve chest tightness, which can often accompany coughing.

To use coriander for coughing, it is important to understand the different forms in which the herb is available. Coriander can be found in the form of seeds, leaves, and oil. The most commonly used forms for treating coughing are coriander tea and oil.

To prepare coriander tea, simply boil a few crushed coriander seeds in a cup of water for about 10 minutes. Strain the mixture and add honey to taste. Drink the tea three times a day to help relieve coughing. Coriander oil can be added to hot water and inhaled to help relieve symptoms.

It is important to note that coriander should not be used as a substitute for medical treatment for persistent or severe coughing. If your cough persists for more than a week, it is recommended that you seek medical attention. Additionally, individuals with certain medical conditions, such as allergies or pregnancy, should consult with their healthcare provider before using coriander. This is a useful herb for relieving coughing due to its anti-inflammatory, expectorant, and antispasmodic properties.

19.          *Cinnamon:*                    Cinnamon,

scientifically known as Cinnamomum cassia, is a commonly used spice in traditional medicine for various health issues, including coughing. One of the main reasons cinnamon is used for coughing is because it contains compounds that help reduce inflammation in the respiratory tract. This reduction in inflammation helps to relieve symptoms such as coughing, chest tightness, and difficulty breathing. Furthermore, cinnamon is also believed to possess expectorant properties, which help to loosen mucus and promote its removal from the respiratory tract. This can help to reduce coughing and prevent the buildup of harmful substances in the respiratory system. Additionally, cinnamon's antispasmodic properties can help to relieve chest tightness, which can often accompany coughing.

In order to use cinnamon for coughing, it is important to understand the different forms in which the spice is available. Cinnamon can be found in the form of sticks, powder, and oil. The most commonly used forms for treating coughing are cinnamon tea and oil.

To prepare cinnamon tea, simply boil a few cinnamon sticks in a cup of water for about 10 minutes. Strain the mixture and add honey to taste. Drink the tea three times a day to help relieve coughing. Cinnamon oil can be added to hot water and inhaled to help relieve symptoms.

It is important to note that cinnamon should not be used as a substitute for medical treatment for persistent or severe coughing. If your cough persists for more than a week, it is recommended that you seek medical attention. Additionally, individuals with certain medical conditions, such as liver disease or allergies, should consult with their healthcare provider before using cinnamon.

20.      *Carom Seeds*: Carom seeds, also known as ajwain, are a commonly used spice in traditional medicine for various health issues, including coughing. Carom seeds are used for coughing because they contain compounds that help reduce inflammation in the respiratory tract. This reduction in inflammation helps to relieve symptoms such as coughing, chest tightness, and difficulty breathing. Furthermore, carom seeds are also believed to possess expectorant properties, which help to loosen mucus and promote its removal from the respiratory tract. This can help to reduce coughing and prevent the buildup of harmful substances in the respiratory system. Additionally, carom seeds' antispasmodic properties can help to relieve chest tightness, which can often accompany coughing.

To use carom seeds for coughing, they can be consumed in various forms, such as tea, decoction, or oil. The most commonly used forms for treating coughing are carom seed tea and oil.

To prepare carom seed tea, simply boil a few carom seeds in a cup of water for about 10 minutes. Strain the mixture and add honey to taste. Drink the tea three times a day to help relieve coughing. Carom seed oil can be added to hot water and inhaled to help relieve symptoms.

It is important to note that carom seeds should not be used as a substitute for medical treatment for persistent or severe coughing. If your cough persists for more than a week, it is recommended that you seek medical attention. Additionally, individuals with certain medical conditions, such as allergies or pregnancy, should consult with their healthcare provider before using carom seeds.

21. ***Elderberry:*** Elderberry, scientifically known as Sambucus nigra, is a commonly used plant in traditional medicine for various health issues, including coughing. Elderberry is used for coughing because it contains compounds that help to boost the immune system, making it easier to fight off infections that can cause coughing. Elderberry is also known to have antiviral properties, which can help to prevent the replication of the viruses that cause upper respiratory infections, such as the common cold. Furthermore, elderberry is believed to

possess expectorant properties, which help to loosen mucus and promote its removal from the respiratory tract. This can help to reduce coughing and prevent the buildup of harmful substances in the respiratory system.

Elderberry is available in various forms, including syrup, capsules, and tea. The most commonly used forms for treating coughing are elderberry syrup and tea.

To prepare elderberry tea, simply add a few dried elderberries to a cup of boiling water. Let the mixture steep for about 10 minutes and then strain. Add honey to taste and drink the tea three times a day to help relieve coughing. Elderberry syrup can be taken by the spoonful or added to tea or water.

It is important to note that elderberry should not be used as a substitute for medical treatment for persistent or severe coughing. If your cough persists for more than a week, it is recommended that you seek medical attention. Additionally, individuals with certain medical conditions, such as diabetes or autoimmune diseases, should consult with their healthcare provider before using elderberry.

22.        *Dill:* Dill, scientifically known as Anethum graveolens, is a commonly used herb in traditional medicine for various health issues, including coughing. The main reason dill is used for coughing is

because it contains compounds that help reduce inflammation in the respiratory tract. This reduction in inflammation helps to relieve symptoms such as coughing, chest tightness, and difficulty breathing. Furthermore, dill is also believed to possess expectorant properties, which help to loosen mucus and promote its removal from the respiratory tract. This can help to reduce coughing and prevent the buildup of harmful substances in the respiratory system. Additionally, dill's antispasmodic properties can help to relieve chest tightness, which can often accompany coughing.

To use dill for coughing, it can be consumed in various forms, such as tea, decoction, or oil. The most commonly used forms for treating coughing are dill tea and oil.

To prepare dill tea, simply boil a few dill leaves in a cup of water for about 10 minutes. Strain the mixture and add honey to taste. Drink the tea three times a day to help relieve coughing. Dill oil can be added to hot water and inhaled to help relieve symptoms.

It is important to note that dill should not be used as a substitute for medical treatment for persistent or severe coughing. If your cough persists for more than a week, it is recommended that you seek medical attention. Additionally, individuals with certain medical conditions, such as allergies or pregnancy, should consult with their healthcare provider before using dill.

23.        *Eucalyptus:*                Eucalyptus,
scientifically known as Eucalyptus globulus,
is a commonly used herb in traditional
medicine for various health issues,
including coughing. Eucalyptus contains
compounds that help to loosen mucus and
promote its removal from the respiratory
tract. This can help to reduce coughing
and prevent the buildup of harmful
substances in the respiratory system.
Furthermore, eucalyptus is also known to
possess antispasmodic properties, which
help to relieve chest tightness, which can
often accompany coughing. Additionally,
eucalyptus is believed to have antibacterial
properties, which can help to prevent
the growth of harmful bacteria in the
respiratory system.

To use eucalyptus for coughing, it can be
consumed in various forms, such as tea, oil, or
inhaled through steam. The most commonly used
forms for treating coughing are eucalyptus oil
and steam inhalation.

To prepare eucalyptus tea, simply boil a few
eucalyptus leaves in a cup of water for about 10
minutes. Strain the mixture and add honey to
taste. Drink the tea three times a day to help
relieve coughing. Eucalyptus oil can be added to
hot water and inhaled to help relieve symptoms.
Simply add a few drops of eucalyptus oil to a bowl

of hot water, cover your head with a towel, and inhale the steam.

It is important to note that eucalyptus should not be used as a substitute for medical treatment for persistent or severe coughing. If your cough persists for more than a week, it is recommended that you seek medical attention. Additionally, individuals with certain medical conditions, such as allergies or pregnancy, should consult with their healthcare provider before using eucalyptus.

24.    *Cumin:* Cumin, scientifically known as Cuminum cyminum, is a commonly used spice in many traditional cuisines around the world. In addition to its culinary uses, cumin has also been used in traditional medicine for various health issues, including coughing. One of the main reasons cumin is used for coughing is because it contains compounds that help to loosen mucus and promote its removal from the respiratory tract. This can help to reduce coughing and prevent the buildup of harmful substances in the respiratory system. Furthermore, cumin is also known to possess antispasmodic properties, which help to relieve chest tightness, which can often accompany coughing. Additionally, cumin is believed to have antibacterial properties, which can help to prevent the growth of harmful bacteria in the respiratory system.

To use cumin for coughing, it can be consumed in various forms, such as tea, oil, or added to food. The most commonly used form for treating coughing is cumin tea.

To prepare cumin tea, simply boil a teaspoon of cumin seeds in a cup of water for about 10 minutes. Strain the mixture and add honey to taste. Drink the tea three times a day to help relieve coughing.

It is important to note that cumin should not be used as a substitute for medical treatment for persistent or severe coughing. If your cough persists for more than a week, it is recommended that you seek medical attention. Additionally, individuals with certain medical conditions, such as allergies or pregnancy, should consult with their healthcare provider before using cumin.

25.      *Lozenge:* Lozenges, also known as cough drops, are small, round, hard candies that dissolve in the mouth and provide relief for various symptoms associated with coughing, such as sore throat and throat irritation. Lozenges typically contain a combination of ingredients that are designed to relieve coughing and provide relief for associated symptoms. For example, menthol is a commonly used ingredient in cough drops. Menthol is a natural mint extract that has a cooling effect on the throat and helps to relieve throat irritation. Additionally,

many lozenges also contain ingredients such as eucalyptus, honey, and lemon, which are known for their expectorant and antibacterial properties. These ingredients can help to loosen mucus and promote its removal from the respiratory tract, reducing coughing and preventing the growth of harmful bacteria.

In order to use lozenges effectively for coughing, it is important to follow the manufacturer's instructions. Typically, lozenges are recommended to be used every two to four hours as needed, or as directed by a healthcare provider. The lozenge should be allowed to dissolve slowly in the mouth and not be chewed or swallowed. Additionally, lozenges should not be used for more than two weeks unless directed by a healthcare provider.

It is important to note that lozenges are not suitable for all individuals. Individuals who are allergic to any of the ingredients in the lozenge should avoid using them. Additionally, lozenges should not be used by individuals who have a history of choking, difficulty swallowing, or by young children who have not yet developed the ability to dissolve lozenges in their mouth.

26.      *Onion:* Onions have been used for centuries as a natural remedy for various ailments, including coughing. Onions contain a high concentration of sulfur compounds, including allicin, which have

been shown to have expectorant properties. These sulfur compounds help to loosen mucus in the respiratory tract, making it easier to remove through coughing. This can reduce coughing and provide relief for associated symptoms such as chest congestion. Additionally, onions have antibacterial properties, which can help to prevent the growth of harmful bacteria in the respiratory tract.

One of the most commonly used methods for using onions for coughing is by consuming raw onions. This can be done by slicing or chopping an onion and eating it as is or by incorporating it into a salad or other dish. Raw onions can also be blended with honey to create a cough syrup, which can be consumed several times a day.

Another method for using onions for coughing is to inhale the vapor from cooked onions. To do this, place a sliced onion in a pot with boiling water and allow it to simmer for several minutes. The vapor from the boiling onion can be inhaled through the nose to provide relief for coughing and chest congestion.

It is important to note that onions can cause heartburn and indigestion in some individuals. Additionally, the strong odor of onions can be unpleasant for some people. As with any natural remedy, it is important to consult with a healthcare provider before using onions for coughing to ensure that it is safe and appropriate for your individual needs.

27.        *Celery:* Celery is a commonly consumed vegetable that is known for its many health benefits, including its ability to provide relief for coughing. Celery contains several compounds that have expectorant properties, including apiol and coumarins. These compounds help to loosen mucus in the respiratory tract, making it easier to remove through coughing. Additionally, celery has anti-inflammatory properties, which can help to reduce inflammation in the respiratory tract and provide relief for coughing and chest congestion.

One of the most commonly used methods for using celery for coughing is by consuming celery juice. To make celery juice, wash and chop several stalks of celery, then blend in a blender or juicer. The juice can be consumed several times a day to provide relief for coughing and chest congestion.

Another method for using celery for coughing is to incorporate it into your diet as a part of your meals. Celery can be added to soups, stews, and salads, or it can be consumed as a snack. Celery can also be blended with other ingredients, such as honey or lemon, to create a cough syrup.

It is important to note that celery can cause allergies in some individuals and may interact with certain medications. As with any natural remedy, it is important to consult with a healthcare provider before using celery for coughing to ensure that it is safe and appropriate for your individual needs.

# CHAPTER 5
## *Twenty Natural and Physical Methods for Coughing*

Natural and physical methods for coughing have gained popularity due to their benefits, such as being safe, effective, affordable, and accessible. Unlike medications, natural methods have no side effects and pose no threat to health. Many methods, such as drinking fluids, using a humidifier, and getting rest, have been proven to be effective in reducing coughing. Additionally, these methods are often less expensive than over-the-counter or prescription medications, making them a more accessible option for those on a tight budget. Furthermore, natural methods can be performed at home without any specialized equipment or medical intervention, making them a convenient option for those with limited time or resources. Lastly, natural methods take a holistic approach to address the root cause of coughing, providing a long-term solution. Utilizing natural and physical methods can help individuals alleviate symptoms, address the root cause, and lead a healthier life.

1. ***Take a hot shower:*** Try taking a hot shower or steamy shower or bath to help relax and clear your airways, and to help loosen phlegm in the lungs and ease coughing. Or

just try taking a warm bath with Epsom salts to help soothe sore muscles and reduce inflammation in the airways. Try sitting in the bathroom with the shower running, or hold a warm, damp towel over your face.

2. *Use a humidifier*: Humidity refers to the amount of moisture present in the air. Maintaining the appropriate level of humidity in the home or office can be important for managing coughing and other respiratory symptoms. When the air is too dry, it can cause the mucous membranes in the airways to become dry and irritated, which can lead to coughing. Dry air can also make it more difficult to expectorate mucus, leading to a build-up of mucus in the airways and an increased likelihood of coughing. Using a humidifier can help to add moisture to the air and can be beneficial for managing coughing. A humidifier can add moisture to the air, which can keep the respiratory tract moist, help to soothe a tickly throat and to loosen phlegm, make it easier to cough up, and help to reduce coughing. Or try using a vaporizer or humidifier in your bedroom at night to help keep the air moist and ease coughing. It's important to note that using a humidifier improperly, such as not cleaning it regularly, can increase the risk of bacterial or fungal growth, which can aggravate respiratory conditions. It's also important to use the humidifier with a proper humidity level, generally between 30-50% humidity,

as too much humidity can cause mold and dust mites to grow, which can also aggravate respiratory conditions.

3. ***Get enough rest:*** When you are tired, your body is less able to fight off infection and inflammation, which can make a cough worse. Getting plenty of rest can help the body to heal and recover from a cough.

4. ***Stay away from irritants:*** Avoiding things that can irritate the respiratory tract, such as tobacco smoke and air pollution or strong perfumes, can help to reduce the production of phlegm, to prevent or reduce coughing. Avoiding things that can dry out your throat such as alcohol and caffeine, to keep the lungs healthy.

5. ***Drink plenty of fluids:*** Staying hydrated can help to thin out mucus, making it easier to cough up, and reduce coughing. You can drink plenty of fluids, such as water, clear broths, frozen water or ice pops, or clear juices. Or try drinking hot liquids, such as tea or soup, to help soothe your throat and ease coughing.

6. ***Wash your hands frequently:*** Washing your hands frequently with soap and water can help to reduce the spread of germs and prevent respiratory infections.

7. ***Avoid contact with sick individuals:*** If you are around someone who is sick, try to keep your distance and avoid close contact to reduce the risk of catching their illness.

8. ***Practice good respiratory hygiene:*** Cover your mouth and nose with a tissue when you cough or sneeze and dispose of the tissue promptly. If you don't have a tissue, cough or sneeze into your elbow to reduce the spread of germs.

9. ***Quit smoking:*** If you smoke, quitting is the single most important thing you can do to improve your lung health.

10. ***Exercise regularly:*** Regular exercise can help to improve cardiovascular fitness and respiratory function.

11. ***Get vaccinated:*** Getting vaccinated against respiratory illnesses, such as the flu, can help to protect your lungs.

12. ***Use air purifiers:*** Using an air purifier can help reduce the concentration of allergens and other irritants in the air, which may help alleviate coughing.

13. ***Propping yourself up:*** When you're sleeping, prop yourself up with an extra pillow or two

so that your head is elevated. This can help to reduce congestion and make it easier for mucus to drain from the lungs, then easy to breathe and cough. Postural drainage is a technique that involves positioning the body in a specific way in order to help drain mucus from the lungs. It involves lying down in different positions that allow gravity to help move the mucus towards the airways, where it can be coughed up or suctioned out.

14. *Use steam therapy:* Steam therapy is a simple and effective technique for relieving coughing by helping to loosen mucus and reduce inflammation in the respiratory tract. It can be done by taking a hot shower, using a humidifier, or by inhaling steam from a bowl of hot water. Boil a pot of water and pour it into a large bowl. Place a towel over your head and lean over the bowl, making sure to keep your face about a foot away from the water to avoid burns. Inhale the steam for about 5-10 minutes, or until the water cools down. You can also add a few drops of essential oils, such as eucalyptus, peppermint, or tea tree, to the water to enhance the therapeutic effect of the steam inhalation. Repeat the process as needed.

15. *Get chest physiotherapy:* Chest physiotherapy, also known as chest physical therapy or postural drainage, involves using

techniques such as clapping or vibrating the chest to help loosen and clear phlegm. Chest physiotherapy technique, such as postural drainage or vibration therapy, to help clear mucus from your lungs and ease coughing.

Chest physiotherapy is a type of treatment that uses various techniques to help clear mucus from the lungs and improve breathing. The two techniques that are commonly used to help ease coughing are postural drainage and vibration therapy.

Chest physiotherapy is usually done under the supervision of a respiratory therapist, physiotherapist, or a nurse. They will teach you how to perform the technique correctly and how to use any equipment if needed.

It's important to note that chest physiotherapy is not suitable for everyone, it is usually recommended for people with chronic lung conditions such as cystic fibrosis, chronic obstructive pulmonary disease (COPD) or bronchiectasis. If you have any of those conditions, it's recommended to consult with your healthcare provider before starting chest physiotherapy.

16. *Use a saline nasal spray:* A saline nasal spray can help to moisten the nasal passages and loosen phlegm in throat, which can reduce the tickle that causes coughing and to ease congestion and cough.

Saline nasal sprays and drops are solutions made from salt and water. They can help to moisten and clear the nasal passages, which can help to reduce congestion and coughing. The salt in the solution helps to break up mucus and clear out the nasal passages. Saline sprays and drops are available over the counter and can be used by both adults and children. They are considered safe and effective for most people.

To use a saline nasal spray, simply tilt your head back and spray the solution into your nostrils, one at a time. To use saline nasal drops, lay down and tilt your head back and place a few drops in each nostril. After using the solution, you can blow your nose to remove any mucus.

It's important to note that if you have any ear, nose or throat condition such as sinusitis, a deviated septum or nasal polyps, please consult with your healthcare provider before using a saline nasal spray, as it may not be suitable for you.

17. *Eat a healthy diet:* A healthy diet that is rich in fruits, vegetables, and whole grains can help to support overall health and lung function.

18. *Use a menthol rub or vapor rub:* These can help to open up the airways and reduce the tickle that causes coughing. Menthol or

eucalyptus chest rub or inhalant to help relieve coughing.

Chest rubs and inhalants are topical medications that contain ingredients such as menthol, eucalyptus, and camphor that help to relieve coughing and congestion. They are applied to the chest and throat, and can be used to help relieve symptoms of colds, flu, and bronchitis. Menthol and eucalyptus are known for their decongestant properties, they can help to open up the airways and make it easier to breathe. Camphor is an anesthetic and a mild anti-inflammatory, it can help to reduce pain and inflammation in the chest and throat.

Chest rubs are typically applied to the skin, while inhalants are meant to be inhaled through the nose or mouth. They can be found in most drugstores, supermarkets, and online as ointments, balms or oils. They are considered safe and effective when used as directed.

It's important to follow the instructions on the product label, and avoid using these products on children under 2 years old, or in case of any allergies to the ingredients. Also, if you have asthma or other respiratory conditions, please consult with your healthcare provider before using these products.

19. *Use chest percussion devices (Vibration therapy)* such as a flutter valve or Acapella, to help clear mucus from your lungs

and ease coughing. Chest percussion is a technique that uses mechanical vibration to help loosen and clear mucus from the lungs. A chest percussion device is a mechanical device that produces vibrations that are directed to the chest, which help to break up and remove mucus from the lungs.

A flutter valve is a small, handheld device that is held against the chest while the person exhales. The vibration causes the mucus in the lungs to loosen and be expelled when the person coughs. The Acapella is a device that uses a vibrating PEP (Positive Expiratory Pressure) technique. It vibrates at high frequency when the patient exhales through it, which helps to break up and move mucus out of the lungs. Chest percussion devices can be used as an adjunct to other treatments, such as postural drainage, vibration therapy, and bronchodilators. They can be used by people with chronic lung conditions such as cystic fibrosis, chronic bronchitis, and chronic obstructive pulmonary disease (COPD).

It's important to note that chest percussion devices should be used under the supervision of a healthcare professional, such as a respiratory therapist, as they can cause discomfort or pain if used incorrectly. Additionally, people with certain medical conditions such as pleural effusion, pneumothorax, or recent chest surgery should consult with their healthcare provider before using these devices.

### 20. Things to avoid if you are coughing:

- Avoid exposure to allergens: If you have allergies, avoiding exposure to allergens such as pollen and pet dander can help reduce coughing.
- Avoid cold drinks: Cold drinks can irritate the throat and worsen coughing.
- Avoid dry air: Dry air can irritate the respiratory system and worsen coughing.
- Avoid any irritating foods that can bother your throat.
- Avoid second-hand smoke: Exposure to second-hand smoke can also irritate the respiratory system and trigger coughing. Avoiding environments where smoking is allowed can help reduce the risk of coughing.
- Avoid allergens: If a cough is triggered by allergies, it can help to avoid exposure to allergens such as pollen, mold, and dust.
- Avoid spicy food: Spicy foods can irritate the throat and make your cough worse.
- Avoid acidic food: Foods that are high in acid, such as citrus fruits and tomatoes, can irritate the throat and make your cough worse.
- Avoid fried food: Fried foods can be difficult to digest and may make your

cough worse.
- Avoid cold air: If cold air triggers your tickly cough, try to stay indoors during cold weather or wear a scarf to cover your nose and mouth.
- Avoid dairy products: Dairy products, such as milk, cheese, and ice cream, can increase mucus production, which can make your cough worse.

Specifically to avoid following:
- Avoid alcohol: Alcohol is a psychoactive substance that can impair immune function and increase the risk of respiratory infections. It can also worsen cough symptoms by dehydrating the body and by irritating the throat and respiratory tract. It is recommended to limit the intake of alcohol and to choose non-alcoholic beverages, such as water, tea, and juice, instead.
- Avoid caffeine. Caffeine is a stimulant that can impair immune function and increase the risk of respiratory infections. It can also worsen cough symptoms by dehydrating the body and by irritating the throat and respiratory tract. It is recommended to limit the intake of caffeine and to choose decaffeinated or caffeine-free beverages, such as water, tea, and juice, instead.
- Avoid refined sugars: Refined sugars,

such as white sugar, brown sugar, and high fructose corn syrup, are highly processed and lack nutritional value. They can weaken immune function, increase inflammation, and increase the risk of respiratory infections. It is recommended to limit the intake of refined sugars and to choose natural sweeteners, such as honey, maple syrup, agave nectar, and molasses, instead.

# CHAPTER 6
## *Traditional Chinese Medicine for Coughing*

Ancient Chinese medical texts describe cough as a symptom of an underlying imbalance or disorder in the body. In traditional Chinese medicine, the lungs and the qi (or life energy) are closely connected, and a cough is often seen as a sign of a problem with the lungs or the qi. The texts also describe different types of coughs, such as dry coughs and productive coughs, and attribute them to different causes and imbalances in the body. Treatment for a cough in traditional Chinese medicine typically involves a combination of herbal medicine, acupuncture, and lifestyle changes to address the underlying cause and bring balance to the body. (This chapter focuses on Chinese herbs, while acupuncture and lifestyle will be discussed in more detail in other chapters.)

***Traditional Chinese Medicine (TCM)*** has a unique approach to diagnosing and treating health conditions, including coughing. In TCM, the clinical differentiation method is used to determine the root cause of the cough and to design an individualized treatment plan. According to TCM, coughing can be classified into various patterns, including exterior wind-cold, wind-heat, interior cold, interior heat, damp-phlegm, dryness, deficiency of qi and yin, and others. The symptoms and patterns of coughing in each individual patient are evaluated through the four diagnostic methods in TCM: inspection, auscultation and olfaction, inquiry, and palpation. Therefore, the clinical differentiation method in TCM provides a holistic approach to diagnosing and treating coughing by considering the individual's unique symptoms and patterns.

> 1.        In TCM, coughing due to *Exterior Wind-Cold* is a common condition that is caused by the invasion of external pathogenic factors, such as wind, cold, and dampness. This type of coughing is characterized by sudden onset, chilliness, body aches, and a thin white tongue coating. Herbal formulas are commonly used in TCM to treat coughing due to exterior wind-cold. These formulas typically contain a combination of herbs that are chosen based on their ability to dispel the pathogenic factors, improve the overall function of the respiratory system, and relieve coughing. Some common herbs used in herbal formulas for this condition include cinnamon, ginger, and ginseng.

One popular herbal formula for treating coughing due to exterior wind-cold is the Gui Zhi Tang formula. This formula consists of cinnamon twigs, ginger, licorice root, and other herbs that are chosen for their ability to dispel the cold, warm the body, and improve the overall function of the respiratory system. The herbs in this formula are combined in specific proportions to produce a synergistic effect, making it a highly effective treatment for coughing due to exterior wind-cold.

Another effective herbal formula for this condition is the Ma Huang Tang formula, which consists of ephedra, ginger, licorice root, and other herbs that are chosen for their ability to dispel the cold, improve the overall function of the respiratory system, and relieve coughing. This formula is particularly useful for treating severe cases of coughing due to exterior wind-cold, as it contains ephedra, which is a potent herb that can effectively dispel the cold and restore the normal flow of qi.

It is important to note that herbal formulas should only be used under the guidance of a licensed practitioner of TCM. This is because the correct diagnosis and treatment of coughing due to exterior wind-cold requires a comprehensive evaluation of the patient's symptoms, including the type and severity of the coughing, the presence of other symptoms, and the patient's overall health status. A licensed practitioner of TCM will be able to design an individualized treatment plan that takes all of these factors into consideration and includes the use of appropriate herbal formulas.

To prevent coughing due to exterior wind-cold, it is important to take measures to protect yourself from external pathogenic factors. This may involve wearing warm clothing, avoiding exposure to wind and dampness, and maintaining a healthy diet. Additionally, it is important to seek prompt treatment if you experience symptoms of coughing, as early treatment can often result in a faster and more complete recovery.

2.           Coughing due to *Exterior Wind-Heat* is typically characterized by symptoms such as a dry or tickling throat, sore throat, headache, and fever. While over-the-counter cough medications can provide temporary relief, they may not address the underlying cause of the cough. Traditional Chinese Medicine (TCM) provides a holistic approach to treating coughs caused by exterior wind-heat. According to TCM, exterior wind-heat is a condition where external factors, such as wind and heat, invade the body and disrupt its natural balance. To treat this type of cough, TCM practitioners may prescribe a herbal formula that works to clear the exterior wind-heat, nourish the lungs, and resolve the underlying imbalance.

One commonly used herbal formula for treating coughing due to exterior wind-heat is the Yin Qiao San formula. This formula contains a combination of herbs that work together to clear exterior wind-heat, relieve throat irritation, and support the immune system. Some of the key ingredients in Yin Qiao San include honeysuckle flowers, forsythia fruit, and lophatherum herb.

Another commonly used formula is the Gui Zhi Tang formula. This formula contains cinnamon twigs, which help to clear exterior wind-heat and promote sweating. Other ingredients in the formula, such as ginger, licorice root, and jujube fruit, work to support the immune system and soothe the throat.

It is important to note that while these herbal formulas can be effective in treating coughing due to exterior wind-heat, they should not be used without the guidance of a licensed practitioner of TCM. Different individuals may have different imbalances and require different formulations, and an experienced practitioner can help determine the most appropriate formula for each individual.

3.          Coughing due to *Interior Cold* is characterized by symptoms such as a congested chest, phlegm, and a tendency to cough more when exposed to cold. According to TCM, interior cold is a condition where the body's natural warmth is obstructed, leading to an accumulation of cold and phlegm in the lungs. To treat this type of cough, TCM practitioners may prescribe a herbal formula that works to dispel the interior cold, resolve the underlying imbalance, and promote the flow of Qi (vital energy).

One commonly used herbal formula for treating coughing due to interior cold is the Gui Zhi Jia Long Gu Mu Li Tang formula. This formula contains a combination of herbs that work together to dispel interior cold, warm the lungs, and promote the flow of Qi. Some of the key ingredients in this formula include cinnamon twigs, dragon bones, deer antler, and oyster shell.

Another commonly used formula is the Ma Xing Shi Gan Tang formula. This formula contains ephedra, ginger, and licorice root, which work to dispel interior cold and warm the lungs. Other ingredients in the formula, such as pinellia tuber and jujube fruit, help to regulate the flow of Qi and support the immune system.

4.          Coughing due to *Interior Heat* is characterized by symptoms such as a dry throat, irritability, and a tendency to cough more in warm or hot environments. Traditional Chinese Medicine (TCM) provides a holistic approach to treating coughs caused by interior heat. According to TCM, interior heat is a condition where there is an excess of heat in the body, leading to symptoms such as a dry throat and coughing. To treat this type of cough, TCM practitioners may prescribe a herbal formula that works to clear the interior heat, nourish the lungs, and resolve the underlying imbalance.

One commonly used herbal formula for

treating coughing due to interior heat is the Yin Qiao San formula. This formula contains a combination of herbs that work together to clear interior heat, relieve throat irritation, and support the immune system. Some of the key ingredients in Yin Qiao San include honeysuckle flowers, forsythia fruit, and lophatherum herb.

Another commonly used formula is the Zhi Bo Di Huang Wan formula. This formula contains rehmannia root, which helps to clear interior heat and nourish the blood. Other ingredients in the formula, such as moutan root and hoelen fungus, work to support the immune system and soothe the throat.

5.          Coughing due to *Damp-Phlegm* is characterized by symptoms such as a congested chest, excessive phlegm, and a tendency to cough more when exposed to damp environments. According to TCM, damp-phlegm is a condition where dampness accumulates in the body, leading to symptoms such as congestion, phlegm production, and coughing. To treat this type of cough, TCM practitioners may prescribe a herbal formula that works to dispel the damp-phlegm, resolve the underlying imbalance, and support the lungs.

One commonly used herbal formula for treating coughing due to damp-phlegm is the Ban Xia Hou Po Tang formula. This formula contains a combination of herbs that work together to dispel damp-phlegm, regulate the spleen, and soothe the throat. Some of the key ingredients in this formula include pinellia tuber, magnolia bark, and dried ginger.

Another commonly used formula is the Wen Dan Tang formula. This formula contains cinnamon twigs, ginger, and licorice root, which work to warm the middle burner and dispel damp-phlegm. Other ingredients in the formula, such as Zhejiang fritillary bulb and ophiopogon root, help to regulate the spleen and support the lungs.

> 6.          Coughing due to **Dryness** is characterized by symptoms such as a dry throat, itching, and a tendency to cough more in dry or windy environments. According to TCM, dryness is a condition where there is a deficiency of moisture in the body, leading to symptoms such as a dry throat, itching, and coughing. To treat this type of cough, TCM practitioners may prescribe a herbal formula that works to moisten the body, nourish the lungs, and resolve the underlying imbalance.

One commonly used herbal formula for treating coughing due to dryness is the Yu Ping Feng San formula. This formula contains a combination of herbs that work together to clear the body of wind, moisten the lungs, and support the immune system. Some of the key ingredients in this formula include magnolia bark, chrysanthemum flower, and the root of the large-leaved gentian.

Another commonly used formula is the Mai Men Dong Tang formula. This formula contains mai men dong root, which helps to moisten the lungs and nourish the body. Other ingredients in the formula, such as ophiopogon root and tangerine peel, work to clear the body of wind and support the immune system.

7.          Coughing can be a symptom of a deeper imbalance in the body, such as a **Deficiency of Qi and Yin**. According to Traditional Chinese Medicine (TCM), qi is the body's vital energy that is responsible for maintaining healthy bodily functions, while yin is the body's vital fluid that provides nourishment and moisture to the body. When there is a deficiency of both qi and yin, it can lead to symptoms such as coughing, fatigue, and a weakened immune system.

To address a deficiency of qi and yin, TCM practitioners may prescribe a herbal formula that works to support the body's energy and fluid levels. One commonly used formula is the Liu Wei Di Huang Wan formula. This formula contains a combination of herbs that work together to nourish the body's yin and support the health of the kidneys, which are believed to be the root of qi and yin in the body according to TCM. Some of the key ingredients in the Liu Wei Di Huang Wan formula include rehmannia root, Chinese yam, and cornus fruit. These herbs work together to nourish the body's yin, support the health of the kidneys, and promote healthy energy levels.

Another commonly used formula for treating a deficiency of qi and yin is the Bu Zhong Yi Qi Wan formula. This formula contains a combination of herbs that work together to support the body's energy and fluid levels, as well as to strengthen the spleen, which is responsible for producing qi in the body according to TCM. Some of the key ingredients in this formula include astragalus root, atractylodes root, and ginger.

It is important to note that while these herbal formulas can be effective in treating a deficiency of qi and yin, they should not be used without the guidance of a licensed practitioner of TCM. Different individuals may have different imbalances and require different formulations, and an experienced practitioner can help determine the most appropriate formula for each individual.

Herbal formulas used to treat a cough in traditional Chinese medicine often include herbs that are expectorant, anti-inflammatory, and immune-boosting. Here is a list of Chinese herbs that are commonly used to treat a cough in traditional Chinese medicine:

**Scutellaria baicalensis (Huang Qin)** - said to clear heat in the lungs and dry dampness.

**Radix Platycodi (Jie Geng)** -said to clear heat and dry dampness, it helps to release the exterior and transform phlegm.

**Radix Glycyrrhizae or Liquorice Root (Gan Cao)** - It helps to regulate the qi and harmonize the lungs. It also has anti-inflammatory properties and helps to reduce phlegm.

**Fructus Schisandrae (Wu Wei Zi)** - It helps to nourish the lungs and strengthen the immune system, also helps to reduce phlegm.

**Fritillariae Thunbergii (Zhe Bei Mu)** -said to clear heat and dry dampness, it helps to release the exterior and transform phlegm.

**Rhizoma Pinelliae (Ban Xia)** - It helps to dry dampness and transform phlegm.

**Radix Stemonae (Bei Qi)** - said to clear heat and dry dampness, it helps to release the exterior and transform phlegm

**Radix Saposhnikoviae (Fang Feng)** - It helps to release the exterior and disperse wind-heat, it also has anti-inflammatory properties.

**Radix Aucklandiae (Mu Xiang)** - It helps to dry dampness and move the qi, it also helps to reduce phlegm.

**Herba Ephedrae (Ma Huang)** - It helps to release the exterior and disperse wind-heat, it's a stimulant and used in small doses.

**Fructus Trichosanthis (Tian Hua Fen)** - It helps to

moisten the lungs and reduce phlegm.

*Rhizoma Atractylodis Macrocephalae (Bai Zhu)* - It helps to dry dampness and strengthen the spleen; it also helps to reduce phlegm.

*Radix Astragali or Astragalus Root (Huang Qi)* - It helps to tonify the qi and strengthen the immune system, it also has anti-inflammatory properties.

*Radix Codonopsis (Dang Shen)* - It helps to tonify the qi and nourish the lungs, it also helps to reduce phlegm.

*Radix Bupleuri (Chai Hu)* - It helps to regulate the qi and release the exterior; it also has anti-inflammatory properties.

*Herba Menthae (Bo He)* - It helps to clear heat and release the exterior; it also has anti-inflammatory properties.

*Flos Lonicerae or Honeysuckle Flower (Jin Yin Hua)* - It helps to clear heat and dry dampness; it also helps to reduce phlegm.

*Rhizoma Zingiberis (Ginger)* - It helps to warm the lungs and release the exterior; it also has anti-inflammatory properties.

Specially recommendation by clinical experience:

*Chuanbei Loquat Syrup (Ninjiom Chuanbei Pipa Gao):* It is suitable for cold and cough, thick phlegm, asthma with phlegm, dry itchy throat, and hoarse voice. This herbal syrup can moisturize the lungs and resolve phlegm, relieve cough and asthma, protect the throat, and relieve the throat. However, children and women who are in their menstrual period or breastfeeding should not use it.

It's important to note that the selection of herbs and the specific formulation of a Chinese herbal formula will depend on the individual case, as different patterns of disharmony will require different combinations of herbs to address the underlying cause of the cough. Also, these herbs should be prepared by a professional experienced in the field. Furthermore, some herbs may interact with other medications or may not be suitable for certain individuals. Therefore, it's always best to consult with a licensed practitioner before taking any herbs.

# CHAPTER 7
## Acupuncture and Acupressure for Coughing

A cupuncture is a form of Traditional Chinese Medicine (TCM) that has been used for thousands of years to treat a wide range of health conditions, including coughing. Acupuncture is based on the principle that a person's health is determined by the balance of energy, or Qi, that flows through the body along pathways known as meridians. By inserting fine, sterile needles into specific points along these meridians, acupuncture can stimulate the body's natural healing response and help to restore balance to the body's energy.

In the treatment of coughing, acupuncture works by regulating the body's energy and improving lung function. According to TCM, coughing can be caused by a number of factors, including internal imbalances, environmental factors, and emotional stress. Acupuncture works to address these underlying causes and improve the overall functioning of the body.

Here is a list of some acupuncture points that are commonly used to treat a cough in traditional Chinese medicine:

- *Lung 7 (LU7) - Called "Lieque"* in Chinese, it is located on the radial side of the wrist, in the depression between the radius and the tendon of the flexor carpi radialis muscle. This point is believed to regulate the body's Qi and help to improve lung function and reduce phlegm.

- *Large Intestine 20 (LI20) - Called "Yingxiang"* in Chinese, it is located on the cheekbone, in the depression directly below the midpoint of the lower border of the orbit. It is said to help clear heat and release the exterior, it's also used to clear nasal congestion.

- *Stomach 36 (ST36) - Called "Zusanli"* in Chinese, it is located on the anterior aspect of the leg, four finger breadths below the kneecap, one finger breadth lateral to the tibia. It is said to help tonify the qi and strengthen the spleen, it's also used as a general tonification point.

- *Pericardium 6 (PC6) - Called "Neiguan"* in Chinese, it is located on the medial aspect of the forearm, three fingerbreadths above the transverse crease of the wrist, in the depression between the tendons of the palmaris longus and the flexor carpi radialis muscles. It is said to help regulate the qi and harmonize the chest, it's also used to alleviate pain and nausea.

- *Conception Vessel 17 (CV17) - Called "Shanzhong"* in Chinese, it is located on the midline of the chest, in the depression between the clavicles, level with the 4th intercostal space. This point is believed to have a calming effect on the body and is used to help regulate the body's Qi, improve lung function and harmonize the chest.

- *Governor Vessel 4 (GV4) - Called "Mingmen"* in Chinese, it is located on the lower back, level with the spinous process of the second lumbar vertebra. It is said to help tonify the yang and strengthen the Kidneys.

- *Gallbladder 34 (GB34) - Called "Yanglingquan"* in Chinese, located in the depression behind the head of the shinbone on the lower leg. Stimulating this point can help relieve coughing, shortness of breath.

- *Gallbladder 41 (GB41) - Called "Zulinqi"* in Chinese, it is located on the lateral side of the foot, in the depression just distal to the head of the fifth metatarsal bone. It is said to help disperse wind and release the exterior, it's also used to alleviate pain and cramps

- *Lung 9 (LU9) - Called "Taiyuan"* in Chinese, it is located on the radial side of the thumb, in the depression between the metacarpal bone and the tendons of the extensor pollicis longus and brevis muscles. It is said to help regulate the lungs and reduce phlegm.

- *Kidney 7 (KI7) - Called "Fuliu"* in Chinese, it is located on the medial aspect of the ankle, in the depression anterior and inferior to the medial malleolus. It is said to help tonify the yin and strengthen the Kidneys, it's also used as a general tonification point.

- *Bladder 34 (BL34) - Called "Yanglingquan"* in Chinese, it is located on the lateral aspect of the leg, in the depression below the head of the fibula. It is said to help regulate the qi and strengthen the Kidneys, it's also used to alleviate pain and cramps.

- *Governing vessel 14 (GV14) - Called "Dazhui"* in Chinese, it is located on the posterior aspect of the neck, at the level of the 7th cervical vertebrae, in the depression below the spinous process. It is said to help regulate the qi and harmonize the chest, it's also used to alleviate pain and stiffness.

- *San Jiao 17 (SJ17) - Called "Shangyingxiang"* in Chinese, it is located on the lateral side of the neck, in the depression below the earlobe. It is said to help clear heat and release the exterior.

- *Conception vessel 12 (CV12) - Called "Zhongwan"* in Chinese, it is located on the midline of the abdomen, level with the tip of the xiphoid process. It is said to help regulate the qi and harmonize the stomach, it's also used to alleviate nausea and vomiting.

- *Spleen 6 (SP6) - Called "Sanyinjiao"* in Chinese, it is located on the medial aspect of the leg, 3 finger widths above the medial malleolus, in the depression between the tibia and the fibula. It is said to help tonify the spleen and regulate the qi.

In addition to these specific points, acupuncture practitioners may also use a combination of other points to help improve the body's overall energy balance and reduce coughing symptoms. For example, they may use points along the spleen and stomach meridians to help improve the body's digestive function and strengthen the immune system, which can help reduce the frequency and severity of coughing. These points are sometimes used in combination with herbal medicine and lifestyle changes to address the underlying cause of the cough and bring balance to the body.

It is important to note that while acupuncture can be an effective treatment for coughing, it is not a substitute for conventional medical treatment and should not be used as the sole treatment for serious or life-threatening conditions. When using acupuncture for coughing, it is important to work with a licensed practitioner who has the training and experience to properly diagnose and treat your condition. The acupuncture point prescription and selection will be tailored to the individual case by a licensed practitioner. And a correct needle technique is crucial for the safety and efficacy of the treatment.

In conclusion, acupuncture is a safe and effective treatment for coughing that works by regulating the body's energy and improving lung function. By targeting specific points along the lung and bronchial meridians, acupuncture can help to reduce coughing symptoms and improve the body's overall health and functioning.

*Acupressure* is a form of traditional Chinese medicine that involves the use of finger pressure on specific points on the body to alleviate various health conditions. It is based on the principles of acupuncture, which is the use of needles to stimulate these same points. Acupressure can be a safe and effective method for treating coughing, as well as other respiratory issues.

The first step in using acupressure to treat coughing is to locate the appropriate pressure points. One commonly used pressure point is Lung 1 (LU 1) "Zhongfu" in Chinese, it is located on the chest, level with the space between the first and second ribs. approximately 1.5-2 inches in the depression below the acromial end of the clavicle. This point regulates Lung Qi and stops cough, stimulates the Lung Qi to descend, disperses fullness in the chest.

Another effective pressure point for coughing is Lung 7 (LU7) "Lieque" in Chinese. it is located on the radial side of the wrist, in the depression between the radius and the tendon of the flexor carpi radialis muscle. This point is also associated with the lung meridian and can regulate the body's Qi and help to improve lung function and reduce phlegm.

Another best pressure point for coughing is Conception Vessel 22 (CV 22) "Tiantu " in Chinese, "Celestial Chimney" in English. It is in the center of the suprasternal fossa, at 5 cun superior to the suprasternal notch. CV 22 is a great point for stopping coughing, and also for everything related to the throat. If you have a sore throat, problems with your voice, or trouble swallowing then this is a good point for treatment.

Additionally, Gallbladder 20 (GB 20) "Fengchi" in Chinese. it is located at the base of the skull, can be used to relieve coughing and other respiratory symptoms.

To perform acupressure on these points, simply apply firm pressure with your thumb or index finger for several minutes, until you feel a sensation of warmth or pressure in the area. You can repeat this process several times a day, as needed, until your symptoms improve.

In conclusion, acupressure can be a safe and effective method for treating coughing and other respiratory issues. By locating and stimulating specific pressure points, acupressure can help to improve respiratory function, reduce coughing, and promote overall well-being. If you are considering using acupressure to treat your symptoms, it is important to consult with a licensed practitioner to ensure the best possible outcome.

# CHAPTER 8
## *Aromatherapy for Coughing*

Aromatherapy is the practice of using essential oils for healing and relaxation. To use essential oils for aromatherapy, you can use a diffuser or a humidifier to disperse the essential oils into the air. You can also inhale the essential oils directly from the bottle or from a tissue, or you can apply them topically to the skin, such as on the chest, neck, or wrists. Some essential oils that may be helpful for cough relief include eucalyptus, peppermint, pine, tea tree, and thyme.

Essential oils are highly concentrated plant extracts that contain the natural aroma and therapeutic properties of the plant. They are extracted from different parts of plants, such as flowers, leaves, stems, roots, and seeds, using a variety of methods, such as steam distillation, cold pressing, or solvent extraction. Essential oils are used for a variety of purposes, including aromatherapy, skincare, and natural remedies.

Essential oils can be used for cough relief due to their antimicrobial, anti-inflammatory, expectorant, and other properties. They can help relieve cough symptoms by reducing inflammation in the respiratory tract, by eliminating or inhibiting the growth of respiratory pathogens, by breaking down and eliminating mucus, and by suppressing cough reflexes. Essential oils can also boost the immune system by providing nutrients, antioxidants, and other beneficial compounds, and by stimulating the production of antibodies. To use essential oils for cough relief, you can try the following methods:

Massage: Massage is the practice of manipulating the soft tissues of the body to promote relaxation and healing. To use essential oils for massage, you can dilute a few drops of the essential oil in a carrier oil, such as almond oil, coconut oil, or olive oil, and apply it to the skin. You can focus on areas of the body that are congested or inflamed, such as the chest, back, or throat. Some essential oils that may be helpful for cough relief include frankincense, ginger, lemon, and rosemary.

Inhalation: Inhalation is the practice of inhaling the aroma of essential oils to promote healing and relaxation. To use essential oils for inhalation, you can use a diffuser or a humidifier to disperse the essential oils into the air, or you can inhale the essential oils directly from the bottle or from a tissue. Some essential oils that may be helpful for cough relief when inhaled include eucalyptus, peppermint, pine, tea tree, and thyme.

Following essential oils can be an effective treatment for coughing:

*Rosemary Essential Oil:* This oil is known for its ability to improve respiratory function and reduce coughing.

**Frankincense Essential Oil:** This oil has been used for centuries to treat respiratory issues, including coughing. It helps to reduce inflammation and improve lung function.

*Eucalyptus Essential Oil:* This oil is well-known for its expectorant properties and is often used to treat respiratory issues, including coughing.

*Peppermint Essential Oil:* This oil contains menthol, which helps to soothe and relax the airways, making it an effective treatment for coughing.

*Thyme Essential Oil:* This oil has antiseptic and expectorant properties that make it an excellent treatment for respiratory issues, including coughing.

*Lemon Essential Oil:* This oil is rich

in antioxidants and has expectorant properties that make it an effective treatment for coughing.

*Ginger Essential Oil:* This oil has anti-inflammatory properties that make it an excellent treatment for coughing and other respiratory issues.

*Lavender Essential Oil:* This oil is known for its calming and relaxing properties, making it an effective treatment for coughing that is caused by stress or anxiety.

*Tea Tree Essential Oil:* This oil has antiseptic and antimicrobial properties that make it an excellent treatment for respiratory infections, including coughing.

*Oregano Essential Oil:* This oil has antiseptic and anti-inflammatory properties that make it an effective treatment for respiratory issues, including coughing

*Clove Essential Oil:* This oil is known for its antiseptic properties and is often used to treat respiratory infections, including coughing.

*Marjoram Essential Oil:* This oil has expectorant properties that make it an effective treatment for coughing.

*Pine Essential Oil:* This oil has expectorant properties that make it an excellent treatment for respiratory issues, including coughing.

*Sandalwood Essential Oil:* This oil is known for its calming properties and is often used to treat respiratory issues, including coughing.

*Basil Essential Oil:* This oil has expectorant properties that make it an effective treatment for coughing.

*Cinnamon Essential Oil:* This oil has antiseptic and anti-inflammatory properties that make it an effective treatment for respiratory issues, including coughing.

*Cypress Essential Oil:* This oil has antiseptic properties and is often used to treat respiratory issues, including coughing.

*Tangerine Essential Oil:* This oil is known for its ability to improve respiratory function and reduce coughing.

*Grapefruit Essential Oil:* This oil is rich

in antioxidants and has expectorant properties that make it an effective treatment for coughing.

***Fennel Essential Oil:*** This oil has antiseptic properties and is often used to treat respiratory issues, including coughing.

It is important to note that essential oils are highly concentrated and should be used with caution. They should be diluted before use and may cause irritation or sensitization when applied to the skin. They should also be avoided by pregnant or nursing women, and by people with certain medical conditions, such as epilepsy, asthma, or allergies. Some essential oils are not safe for certain individuals, such children, and can cause adverse reactions if used improperly. Additionally, some essential oils should not be taken internally and should only be used topically or through inhalation. It is recommended to consult with a healthcare professional or a certified aromatherapist before using essential oils for cough relief.

# CHAPTER 9

## *Food Therpies for Coughing*

F ood therapy is an important aspect of traditional Chinese medicine, and it can be used to help alleviate a variety of health conditions, including coughing. Fruits and vegetables that are high in vitamin C, such as oranges, lemons, and berries, can help to boost the immune system and reduce inflammation in the airways, which can help to relieve coughing.

Nutrition plays a crucial role in maintaining overall health and can also be an effective tool for managing coughing. A well-balanced diet that includes a variety of nutrient-dense foods can support the body's natural healing processes, reduce inflammation, and promote optimal respiratory function. Anti-inflammatory foods are particularly beneficial for managing coughing. Inflammation in the airways is a common cause of coughing and other respiratory symptoms. Consuming foods that have anti-inflammatory properties can help to reduce inflammation in the airways, which can in turn reduce coughing.

Some fresh fruits and vegetables are rich in antioxidants, vitamins, and minerals that can help to reduce inflammation in the body. Berries, leafy greens, and cruciferous vegetables are particularly high in anti-inflammatory compounds. Omega-3 fatty acids are healthy fats, which can be found in foods such as fish, flaxseed, and chia seeds, can help to reduce inflammation throughout the body, including the airways. A lot of spices and herbs such as ginger, turmeric, and garlic, have anti-inflammatory properties. Most whole grains are rich in fiber, vitamins, and minerals, which can help to reduce inflammation in the body. Probiotics are also very good. Foods such as yogurt, kefir, kimchi, and sauerkraut contain probiotics, which can help to improve gut health and reduce inflammation throughout the body.

Here is a list of foods that can help to relieve coughing:

- **Oranges**: Oranges are a rich source of vitamin C, which can help to boost the immune system and reduce inflammation in the airways. Try drinking a glass of fresh orange juice or eating an orange as a snack.

- **Lemons**: Lemons are another great source of vitamin C, and they can also help to soothe a sore throat and reduce inflammation in the airways. Try drinking a glass of warm water with lemon and honey or add a squeeze of fresh lemon juice into warm water or tea to help reduce coughing.

- **Berries:** Berries, such as strawberries, raspberries, and blueberries, are also high in vitamin C, as well as other antioxidants. They can help to boost the immune system and reduce inflammation in the airways. They can be eaten fresh or frozen and can be added to smoothies or yogurt.

- **Papaya:** Papaya is a great source of vitamin C and contains enzymes called papain and chymopapain that can help to break down mucus and reduce inflammation in the airways.

- **Kiwi:** Kiwi is another good source of vitamin C and contains potassium and vitamin E, both of which help to reduce inflammation in the airways.

- **Guava:** Guava is one of the most Vitamin C rich fruits, it contains four times the Vitamin C of an orange.

- **Ginger:** Ginger is a spice that has been used for centuries to treat coughs and other respiratory conditions. It has anti-inflammatory, expectorant, and antiviral properties that can help relieve cough symptoms and boost the immune system. Ginger can be consumed in various forms, such as fresh ginger root, dried ginger, ginger tea, or ginger supplements. To use ginger for cough relief, you can try the following:

    1. **Fresh ginger root:** Grate or slice a small piece of fresh ginger root and add it to a cup of hot water. Let it steep for 5-10

minutes, then strain and drink. You can sweeten it with honey or another natural sweetener if desired. You can drink ginger tea 2-3 times a day as needed.

2. *Dried ginger:* Add a teaspoon of dried ginger to a cup of hot water. Let it steep for 5-10 minutes, then strain and drink. You can sweeten it with honey or another natural sweetener if desired. You can drink ginger tea 2-3 times a day as needed.

3. *Ginger supplements:* You can also take ginger supplements, such as ginger capsules or ginger extract, according to the instructions on the label. It is important to follow the recommended dosage and to consult with a healthcare professional.

- *Carrot:* Carrots are high in vitamins and minerals, and they can help to soothe the throat and reduce coughing.

- *Spinach:* Spinach is high in vitamins and minerals, and it can help to soothe the throat and reduce coughing.

- *Fennel:* Fennel has natural expectorant properties, and it can help to break up mucus and relieve coughing.

- *Red pepper:* Red pepper contains capsaicin, which can help to soothe the throat and reduce coughing.

- **Lotus root:** Lotus root has natural expectorant properties, and it can help to break up mucus and relieve coughing.

- **Almonds:** Almonds are high in vitamins and minerals, and they can help to soothe the throat and reduce coughing.

- **Sesame seeds:** Sesame seeds are high in vitamins and minerals, and they can help to soothe the throat and reduce coughing.

- **Soybeans:** Soybeans are high in vitamins and minerals, and they can help to soothe the throat and reduce coughing.

- **Chestnuts:** Chestnuts are high in vitamins and minerals, and they can help to soothe the throat and reduce coughing.

- **Sweet potato:** Sweet potatoes are high in vitamins and minerals, and they can help to soothe the throat and reduce coughing.

- **Lotus seeds:** Lotus seeds are high in vitamins and minerals, and they can help to soothe the throat and reduce coughing.

- **Rice:** Rice can help to soothe the throat and reduce coughing, and it is also an important source of energy for the body.

- **Green tea:** Green tea has natural antibacterial and antiviral properties, and it can help to soothe the throat and reduce coughing.

- **Nutmeg:** Nutmeg has natural expectorant

properties, and it can help to break up mucus and relieve coughing.

- **Sage:** Sage has natural expectorant properties, and it can help to break up mucus and relieve coughing.

- **Thyme:** Thyme has natural expectorant properties, and it can help to break up mucus and relieve coughing.

- **Rose hips:** Rose hips are high in vitamins and minerals, and they can help to soothe the throat and reduce coughing.

**Natural sweeteners,** such as maple syrup, agave nectar, and molasses, have been used for centuries as sweeteners and as remedies for a variety of ailments, including coughs. These sweeteners are considered natural because they are derived from plants and are minimally processed. They are often used as alternatives to refined sugar, which is derived from sugar cane or sugar beets and is highly processed, as they are perceived to have more nutritional value and fewer negative health effects.

- **Maple syrup** is a sweet syrup produced from the sap of maple trees. It contains a variety of nutrients, such as carbohydrates, minerals, and vitamins, as well as antioxidants and other beneficial compounds. Maple syrup has been used for centuries as a natural sweetener and as a remedy for a variety of ailments, including coughs. It is believed to have antimicrobial and anti-inflammatory properties that can help relieve cough symptoms and support respiratory health. Maple syrup can be consumed on its own or added to teas, syrups, and other remedies to sweeten and enhance their flavor and effectiveness.

■ *Agave nectar* is a sweet syrup produced from the sap of agave plants. It contains a variety of nutrients, such as carbohydrates, minerals, and vitamins, as well as antioxidants and other beneficial compounds. Agave nectar has been used for centuries as a natural sweetener and as a remedy for a variety of ailments, including coughs. It is believed to have antimicrobial and anti-inflammatory properties that can help relieve cough symptoms and support respiratory health. Agave nectar can be consumed on its own or added to teas, syrups, and other remedies to sweeten and enhance their flavor and effectiveness.

■ *Molasses* is a sweet syrup produced from the juice of sugar cane or sugar beets. It contains a variety of nutrients, such as carbohydrates, minerals, and vitamins, as well as antioxidants and other beneficial compounds. Molasses has been used for centuries as a natural sweetener and as a remedy for a variety of ailments, including coughs. It is believed to have antimicrobial and anti-inflammatory properties that can help relieve cough symptoms and support respiratory health. Molasses can be consumed on its own or added to teas.

It's important to note that getting enough vitamin C through foods is always better than getting it through supplements. Additionally, it's important to vary your diet, and to include a variety of different fruits and vegetables, as well as other nutritious foods, such as lean proteins, whole grains, and healthy fats, to ensure that you're getting all the nutrients you need for optimal health.

We should remember that food therapy should not be used as a sole treatment for coughing, and it should be used in conjunction with other treatments, such as medications and lifestyle changes, to achieve the best possible outcome. You should consider other factors that may be contributing to your coughing, such as allergies, infections, or underlying medical conditions, and seek appropriate medical treatment as needed. Additionally, it is always best to seek the advice of a licensed practitioner before making any changes to your diet or lifestyle.

# CHAPTER 10

## *Over-The-Counter (OTC) Medications for Coughing*

Coughing can be a symptom of many conditions, and there are many over-the-counter (OTC) medications available to help manage it. These medications can be broadly categorized into three types: decongestants, expectorants, and antihistamines. Over-the-counter medications help relieve coughing.

- *Decongestants:* over-the-counter anti-inflammatory medication help reduce inflammation in the airways and ease coughing. These medications are designed to help relieve nasal congestion and can be helpful for managing coughing caused by colds, flu, and other respiratory infections. Decongestants can come in the form of nasal sprays or oral tablets. They work by narrowing the blood vessels in the nasal passages, which reduces inflammation and swelling and allows for easier breathing. Examples of decongestant medications include pseudoephedrine and phenylephrine.

- *Ibuprofen (Advil)* works by reducing

inflammation in the body. When the airways become inflamed, it can cause symptoms such as coughing, chest tightness, and difficulty breathing. By reducing inflammation, anti-inflammatory medications can help to relieve these symptoms. Ibuprofen is a non-steroidal anti-inflammatory drug (NSAID) that is available over-the-counter in various forms such as tablets, capsules, and liquids. It can help to relieve pain and reduce inflammation in the body. It can also be used to help reduce a fever.

It's important to note that anti-inflammatory medications such as ibuprofen may cause side effects such as stomach upset, nausea, and heartburn. They may also interact with other medications you're taking. Also, it's not recommended for children under 6 years old and people with a history of stomach or intestinal ulcers, asthma, bleeding disorders or hypertension. Therefore, it's recommended to consult with your healthcare provider before taking ibuprofen or any other anti-inflammatory medication.


- *Antihistamines:* An antihistamine is a medication that works by blocking the action of histamine, a chemical that is released by the body during an allergic reaction. When histamine is released, it can cause symptoms such as itching, sneezing, runny nose, watery eyes, and coughing. Antihistamines can help to reduce these symptoms and provide relief. They can also be used to manage coughing caused by postnasal drip, a condition in which mucus drips down the back of the throat. Antihistamines can come in the form of tablets, syrups, or nasal sprays. They work by blocking the action of histamine, a chemical that causes inflammation and swelling in the airways. Examples of antihistamine medications include *diphenhydramine, loratadine, and cetirizine.*

· *Diphenhydramine (Benadryl and Tylenol PM)* is one of the most common over-the-counter antihistamines. It is available in tablets, capsules, and liquid forms. Diphenhydramine can help to relieve symptoms of allergic rhinitis, such as runny nose, sneezing, and coughing. It can also help to relieve symptoms of hay fever and other allergies.

It's important to note that Diphenhydramine may cause drowsiness, so it's not recommended to drive or operate heavy machinery after taking it. It's also not recommended for individuals with liver or kidney disease or those taking this medication with alcohol or other sedative medications. Additionally, it's not recommended for children under 2 years old, and consult with your healthcare provider before taking this medication, especially if you have any medical conditions or are taking other medications.

Additionally, *loratadine and cetirizine* should not be used to treat cough caused by a bacterial or viral infection, as they do not have any antimicrobial properties. Also, it is essential to follow the recommended dosage and not exceed the maximum recommended dose, as taking too much of these medications can cause adverse effects.

- *Expectorants*: over-the-counter expectorants help loosen mucus in the airways and make it easier to cough up. Expectorants can come in the form of syrups, capsules, or tablets. They work by increasing the amount of mucus produced in the airways and by making it thinner, allowing it to be coughed up more easily. Examples of expectorant medications include guaifenesin and terpin hydrate.

*Guaifenesin* is a common over-the-counter expectorant that is used to relieve chest congestion caused by colds, flu, and other respiratory conditions. Expectorants are medications that help to loosen and expel mucus from the lungs by increasing the amount of water in the lungs. This makes it easier for the person to cough up and remove the mucus.

Guaifenesin is available in various forms such as tablets, capsules, syrups, liquids and gel form and can be found in several cough and cold remedies such as *Mucinex and Robitussin.* It is considered safe and effective when used as directed. It's usually recommended to take it with a glass of water, and it's not recommended for it's not recommended for children under 6 years old and people with certain medical conditions such as asthma, heart disease, high blood pressure or kidney problems, or those taking certain medications such as cough suppressants or decongestants, because they may have opposite effects.

- *Dextromethorphan (DXM or DM)* is a cough suppressant that works by suppressing the cough reflex in the brain. It is available in syrup, capsule, and lozenge form and can be found in several cough and cold remedies such as **Robitussin, Vicks Formula 44, and Nyquil.** Dextromethorphan is considered safe for most people, but it is not recommended for individuals with liver or kidney disease, or those taking certain medications.

- **Mucolytics** are medications that help break down and thin mucus in the respiratory tract, making it easier to cough up. They are available in syrup and tablet form and can be found in several cough and cold remedies such as **Mucinex and Bromhexine.** Mucolytics are considered safe for most people but may cause stomach upset in some individuals.

- *Menthol* is a natural ingredient that has a cooling and soothing effect on the respiratory tract, making it an effective cough suppressant. It is available in lozenge, gel, and oil form and can be found in several cough and cold remedies such as **Halls and Vicks VapoRub**. Menthol is considered safe for most people but may cause skin irritation in some individuals.

It is important to note that OTC cough and cold remedies are not recommended for individuals under the age of 2, and they should be used with caution in children under the age of 6. Also, it is essential to follow the recommended dosage and not exceed the maximum recommended dose, as taking too much of these medications can be harmful.

# CHAPTER 11
## Yoga, Tai Chi, Qigong and Exercises for Coughing

**Y**oga is a practice that combines physical postures, breathing techniques, and meditation, and has been found to be beneficial for a wide range of health conditions, including respiratory conditions. Some studies have found that regular yoga practice can help to reduce the frequency and severity of coughing and improve lung function in people with respiratory conditions such as asthma and COPD. This may be due to the combination of deep breathing, body postures, and relaxation techniques used in yoga, which can help to open up the airways and make it easier to cough up mucus.

Yoga and breathing exercises are natural methods to alleviate coughing and improve overall respiratory function. Yoga poses, such as forward bends and twists, can help to open up the chest and lungs, allowing for better airflow and reducing coughing.

- *Pranayama:* a type of yoga breathing, is specifically designed to improve lung function and promote deep, full breaths. Techniques such as alternate nostril breathing, ujjayi breath, and Kapalabhati can help to clear mucus, reduce inflammation, and relax the respiratory muscles.

- *"Cat-cow" pose:* a specific yoga pose for cough relief is the "cat-cow" pose. This pose involves moving the spine and ribcage in a gentle, back-and-forth motion, which can help to loosen up any congestion and stimulate the lungs.

- *The "child's pose":* it is another yoga pose that can help with coughing by opening up the chest and lungs, allowing for better breathing.

- *The "bridge pose":* it is also effective for coughing, as it opens up the chest and lungs, stretches the shoulders, and strengthens the back muscles.

- *"Fish pose" and "Shoulder stand":* they are also beneficial for respiratory health and are said to help open up the chest and lungs, and to ease breathing.

Yoga and breathing exercises can be done at home, making them easily accessible for people of all ages and abilities. Regular practice of yoga and breathing exercises can help to prevent coughing from recurring by keeping the respiratory system strong and healthy. Yoga and breathing exercises are also considered safe and effective options for pregnant women and children. Yoga and breathing exercises can be used in conjunction with other treatments, such as medication and lifestyle changes, to provide a comprehensive approach to treating coughing. Yoga and breathing exercises are relatively low-cost and do not have any serious side effects. Practicing yoga and breathing exercises can also improve overall wellbeing, by reducing stress and promoting relaxation. Yoga and breathing exercises can be tailored to individual needs, making them an excellent alternative to traditional medications for coughing and respiratory conditions.

It is important to note that Yoga can be adapted to different levels of physical fitness and health conditions, so it is best to consult with a yoga therapist or experienced yoga teacher to find the best practice for you. Yoga should be safe for most people, but as with any form of exercise, it's important to check with your doctor before starting a yoga practice, especially if you have an underlying medical condition or if you are experiencing difficulty breathing.

*Tai Chi* is a traditional Chinese martial art that combines slow, flowing movements with deep breathing and meditation techniques. It is believed to help balance the body's energy, promote physical and mental well-being, and improve overall health. In terms of treating coughing, Tai Chi exercises are designed to help clear mucus from the lungs, improve lung function, and reduce inflammation. Tai Chi may help to reduce the frequency and severity of coughing and improve overall lung function in people with respiratory conditions such as COPD. This is thought to be due to a combination of the gentle movements, breathing techniques, and relaxation practices used in Tai Chi. Some of the specific Tai Chi exercises that may be helpful for coughing include:

- **Deep breathing:** Tai Chi includes deep breathing exercises that focus on expanding the diaphragm, which can help to clear mucus from the lungs.

- **Slow and gentle movements:** Tai Chi exercises are performed slowly and gently, which can help to improve lung function and reduce coughing.

- **Visualization:** Tai Chi includes visualization techniques that can help to reduce stress and improve overall well-being, which can also help to reduce coughing.

- **Some Tai Chi forms include Qigong** exercises that are designed to help improve lung function, reduce inflammation, and reduce coughing in patients with asthma and COPD.

A study published in the Journal of Alternative and Complementary Medicine found that Tai Chi improved lung function and reduced coughing in patients with chronic obstructive pulmonary disease (COPD). Another study published in the Journal of Asthma found that Tai Chi improved lung function and reduced coughing in patients with asthma.

It is important to note that Tai Chi is a low-impact form of exercise and should be safe for most people. However, as with any form of exercise, it's important to check with your doctor before starting a Tai Chi practice, especially if you have an underlying medical condition or if you are experiencing difficulty breathing. Tai Chi is also a form of martial art, and some specific movements and postures can be hard for some people with some medical conditions. So, it is always recommended to consult with an experienced practitioner and get guidance that is tailored to your specific needs.

*Qigong* is a traditional Chinese healing practice that combines movement, breathing, and meditation techniques. It is believed to help balance the body's energy and promote physical and mental well-being. Qigong is a holistic practice that includes physical postures, breathing techniques, and meditation. Qigong exercises for coughing typically involve deep breathing techniques, gentle movements, and visualization. The exercises are designed to help clear mucus from the lungs, improve lung function, and reduce inflammation. Some of the specific Qigong exercises that may be helpful for coughing include:

- *Diaphragmatic breathing:* diaphragmatic breathing can help to clear mucus from the lungs and improve lung function. This technique involves breathing deeply into the diaphragm rather than shallowly into the chest. To do diaphragmatic breathing, you can place one hand on your chest and the other on your stomach and focus on making the hand on your stomach rise while you inhale, while the hand on your chest should remain relatively still. Once you become comfortable with diaphragmatic breathing, you can try to incorporate it into your daily routine to help clear your lungs and reduce coughing.

- **Qi Gong for lungs:** This exercise is designed to help open and clear the lungs, improve breathing, and reduce coughing.

- **Qigong for bronchitis:** This exercise is designed to help clear mucus from the lungs, improve lung function, and reduce inflammation in the bronchial tubes.

- **Qigong for asthma:** This exercise is designed to help improve lung function, reduce inflammation, and reduce coughing in patients with asthma.

There is some evidence to suggest that Qigong may be effective in treating coughing. A study published in the Journal of Traditional Chinese Medicine found that Qigong exercises improved lung function and reduced coughing in patients with chronic obstructive pulmonary disease (COPD). Another study published in the Journal of Clinical Rehabilitation found that Qigong exercises improved lung function and reduced coughing in patients with asthma. It's important to note that Qigong should be performed under the guidance of a qualified Qigong instructor, and it should not be used as a substitute for conventional medical treatment. Qigong may be effective in treating coughing, it should not be used as a substitute for conventional medical treatment.

It's always best to consult with a healthcare professional before trying Qigong or any other alternative therapy.

*Other Exercises* good for coughing:

- *Cardio exercises* such as walking, jogging, cycling or swimming are great for overall lung health and help the body fight off infections. These activities increase the amount of oxygen in your body, which can help to reduce inflammation and open up the airways. It's also important to start with low-impact exercise and gradually increase the intensity as you get stronger.

- *Strength training* is also beneficial for people with a cough as it help to improve the body's ability to fight off infections, and to increase muscle mass, which can help to improve breathing function and reduce symptoms of coughing.

- *Pulmonary rehabilitation* is a program of breathing and physical exercise that can help to improve lung function, reduce symptoms, and improve overall quality of life for people with lung conditions such as COPD. This type of rehabilitation usually includes a combination of breathing exercises, strength training, and endurance exercises, and is usually supervised by a respiratory therapist or other qualified professional.

- *Aerobic exercise:* Engaging in regular aerobic exercise, such as walking, running, or cycling, can help improve lung function and respiratory endurance. This can be especially beneficial for people with conditions such as asthma or COPD.

- *Progressive muscle relaxation:* Progressive muscle relaxation is a technique that involves tensing and then relaxing different muscle groups in the body. It can help to reduce coughing by reducing stress and tension, which can make coughing worse. Progressive muscle relaxation can also help to improve overall relaxation and sleep quality.

- *Guided imagery:* Guided imagery is a technique that involves using the imagination to visualize calming and peaceful scenes. It can help to reduce coughing by reducing stress and tension, which can make coughing worse. Guided imagery can also help to improve overall relaxation and sleep quality.

- *Mindfulness meditation:* Mindfulness meditation is a technique that involves focusing on the present moment and accepting it without judgment. It can help to reduce coughing by reducing stress and tension, which can make coughing worse. Mindfulness meditation can also help to improve overall relaxation and sleep quality.

- *Cognitive behavioral therapy (CBT):* CBT is a form of therapy that focuses on changing negative thought patterns and behaviors. It can help to reduce coughing by reducing stress and tension, which can make coughing worse. CBT can also help to improve overall relaxation and sleep quality.

- *Resistance training:* Resistance training, such as weightlifting, can help improve overall muscle strength, including the muscles used for breathing.

It is always recommended to check with your doctor before starting an exercise program, especially if you have an underlying medical condition, or if you are experiencing difficulty breathing. Additionally, it's important to listen to your body and not push yourself too hard; if you feel pain or discomfort during exercise, stop and consult your doctor.

# CHAPTER 12
## Lifestyle Changes for Coughing

L ifestyle changes can play a significant role in reducing coughing and improving respiratory health. Regular exercise and good posture can help improve respiratory function, reduce coughing, and prevent respiratory problems. By reducing exposure to irritants, such as dust, chemicals, and pollutants, the respiratory system can be protected and coughing can be reduced. A healthy diet, proper hydration, and adequate sleep can help support the immune system, reducing the likelihood of infections that can cause coughing. Reducing stress can have a positive impact on overall health, including respiratory health, and reduce the likelihood of coughing. By maintaining a clean home and using a vacuum with a HEPA filter, the amount of irritants in the environment can be reduced, leading to a reduction in coughing. By seeking medical attention and managing allergies, underlying conditions that can cause coughing can be treated, reducing coughing and improving respiratory health. Implementing these changes can help reduce coughing, prevent respiratory problems, and promote overall health.

- *Staying Hydrated:* Staying hydrated is essential for maintaining overall health and can also play a role in managing coughing. When the body is dehydrated, it can lead to a dryness of the mucous membranes, which line the airways, nose, and throat. These dry membranes can lead to coughing, as the body's natural response to remove the dryness is to cough. By keeping the body hydrated, it can help to keep the mucous membranes moist, reducing the likelihood of coughing. Adequate hydration can also help to keep the mucus in the lungs thin and easier to expectorate, which can reduce the need to cough in order to remove the mucus.

Drinking warm liquids such as tea and water can also be beneficial for managing coughing. Warm liquids can help to soothe the airways and loosen up mucus, making it easier to cough up. The heat from the warm liquids can also stimulate the production of mucus in the airways and sinuses, which can help to clear out any irritants that may be causing the coughing. Additionally, warm liquids can also help to hydrate the body, so they can be an effective way to manage both dryness and coughing.

It's important to note that drinking cold liquids or consuming ice-cold foods can cause the opposite effect and make coughing worse, as they can cause the airways to constrict. Cold liquids can also cause the mucus in the airways to thicken, making it more difficult to expectorate and leading to more coughing.

When it comes to hydration, it's important to aim for at least 8 glasses of water per day, or more if you are active or sweating a lot. You can also include other fluids such as tea, juice, or clear broths to reach your fluid intake goal. Herbal teas, such as ginger, chamomile, or licorice can be particularly soothing for the throat and can help to reduce coughing. It's also important to note that some medications can cause dryness in the mouth, making it important to drink more water and other fluids to prevent this side effect.

Overall, staying hydrated is an important aspect of managing coughing and a simple step that can be easily incorporated into daily routine. It can also be beneficial to drink fluids throughout the day, rather than chugging a lot at once, to keep a steady hydration level. Drinking fluids before bed can also help to prevent dryness and coughing during the night.

- ***Quit Smoking*** is an important step to stop coughing because smoking cigarettes is one of the most common causes of chronic coughing. The chemicals in cigarettes and other tobacco products can irritate the airways and lead to coughing. Smoking can also increase the risk of developing lung cancer, emphysema, and other serious respiratory conditions. If you smoke, quitting is one of the most effective ways to reduce coughing and improve your overall health. Your doctor can provide you with resources and support to help you quit smoking, such as nicotine replacement therapy, medication and counseling.

- **Reducing Air Pollution Exposure:** Air pollution is another common cause of coughing. Exposure to pollutants such as smog, dust, and chemicals can irritate the airways and lead to coughing. In some cases, air pollution can also aggravate pre-existing respiratory conditions such as asthma. If you live in an area with high levels of pollution, it's important to take steps to protect yourself. This can include staying indoors when pollution levels are high, using an air purifier, and wearing a mask when you're outside.

- **Improving Indoor Air Quality** can also be a cause of coughing. Common sources of indoor air pollution include mold, pet dander, dust mites, and cleaning products. To improve indoor air quality, it's important to keep your home clean and well-ventilated, use natural cleaning products, and reduce the number of dust-collecting items in your home. This means frequently cleaning surfaces, carpets, and upholstery, vacuuming, and dusting frequently, and maintaining a proper humidity level.

- **Getting Regular Exercise:** Exercise helps to improve respiratory function and can reduce coughing by promoting good circulation and strengthening the lungs.

- **Getting Adequate Sleep:** Sleep is important for overall health, including respiratory health, and a lack of sleep can increase coughing.

- *Reducing Stress:* Stress can trigger coughing, and reducing stress through relaxation techniques, such as yoga or meditation, can help minimize coughing.

- *Eating a Healthy Diet:* A balanced diet with plenty of fruits and vegetables can provide the nutrients needed to support respiratory health and reduce coughing.

- *Avoiding Irritants:* Certain irritants, such as strong perfumes, chemical fumes, and pet dander, can trigger coughing. Avoiding these triggers can help minimize coughing.

- *Seeking Medical Attention*: If coughing persists or is accompanied by other symptoms, seeking medical attention is important to determine the underlying cause and receive proper treatment.

- *Managing Allergies:* Allergies can cause coughing and other respiratory symptoms, managing allergies through medication, immunotherapy, or avoiding triggers can help reduce coughing.

- *Staying Warm*: Cold air can irritate the respiratory system and trigger coughing, staying warm by wearing a scarf or using a heating blanket can help minimize coughing.

- ***Practicing Good Posture:*** Good posture can help promote proper breathing and reduce coughing.

- ***Maintaining a Clean Home:*** A clean home can reduce the amount of dust and other irritants that can trigger coughing.

# CHAPTER 13

## Massage, Chiropractic and Tui Na Therapy for Coughing

**M**assage therapy is a form of alternative medicine that has been used for centuries to treat a variety of physical and mental conditions. Massage therapy involves the manipulation of soft tissue to improve overall health and well-being. While it is typically used to relieve muscle tension and improve circulation, massage therapy can also be an effective treatment for coughing. Coughing is a common symptom of many conditions, including colds, flu, bronchitis, asthma, and even allergies. It is the body's natural response to remove irritants from the airways. However, in some cases, coughing can become chronic and interfere with daily life. Massage therapy can help alleviate coughing by addressing the underlying causes.

Massage therapy can improve coughing by reducing tension in the muscles that control breathing. When the muscles are tense, they can put pressure on the airways, leading to coughing. Massage therapy can help relieve this tension and improve overall respiratory function. In addition to reducing tension in the muscles, massage therapy can also improve circulation. Improved circulation can help the body remove irritants from the airways more effectively, reducing the likelihood of coughing. Massage therapy can also improve breathing by reducing stress and anxiety. Stress and anxiety can lead to shallow breathing, which can increase the likelihood of coughing. Massage therapy can help relax the body and reduce stress, leading to deeper and more effective breathing.

There are a variety of massage therapy techniques that can be used to treat coughing. These may include Swedish massage, deep tissue massage, and trigger point therapy. Your massage therapist will work with you to determine the best technique for your individual needs.

- *Swedish massage* is a type of therapeutic massage that is designed to promote relaxation, reduce stress and tension, and improve circulation. It is one of the most commonly used forms of massage therapy and is known for its long, smooth strokes, kneading, and friction techniques. While Swedish massage is typically used to relieve muscle tension and promote relaxation, it can also be an effective treatment for coughing.

Swedish massage can help improve coughing by reducing tension in the muscles that control breathing. When the muscles are tense, they can put pressure on the airways, leading to coughing. Swedish massage can help relieve this tension and improve overall respiratory function. In addition to reducing tension in the muscles, Swedish massage can also improve circulation. Improved circulation can help the body remove irritants from the airways more effectively, reducing the likelihood of coughing. Swedish massage can also promote relaxation, which can help reduce stress and anxiety. Stress and anxiety can lead to shallow breathing, which can increase the likelihood of coughing.

Swedish massage is performed using long, smooth strokes, kneading, and friction techniques. Your massage therapist will work with you to determine the best techniques for your individual needs. The massage may also incorporate other forms of therapy, such as aromatherapy, to help promote relaxation and improve overall health and well-being.

- *Deep tissue massage* is a type of therapeutic massage that is designed to relieve tension and pain in the deep layers of muscle and connective tissue. It is a more intense form of massage therapy that is used to address specific areas of tension and discomfort in the body. While deep tissue massage is typically used to relieve muscle pain and improve posture, it can also be an effective treatment for coughing. Deep tissue massage can help improve coughing by reducing tension in the muscles that control breathing. When the muscles are tense, they can put pressure on the airways, leading to coughing. Deep tissue massage can help relieve this tension and improve overall respiratory function. In addition to reducing tension in the muscles, deep tissue massage can also improve circulation. Improved circulation can help the body remove irritants from the airways more effectively, reducing the likelihood of coughing. Deep tissue massage can also promote relaxation, which can help reduce stress and anxiety. Stress and anxiety can lead to shallow breathing, which can increase the likelihood of coughing.

Deep tissue massage is performed using deep, focused pressure and slow strokes to reach the deeper layers of muscle and connective tissue. Your massage therapist will work with you to determine the best techniques for your individual needs. The massage may also incorporate other forms of therapy, such as aromatherapy, to help promote relaxation and improve overall health and well-being.

- *Trigger point massage* is a type of therapeutic massage that focuses on the release of tension in specific areas of the body known as trigger points. These trigger points are tight knots of muscle fibers that can cause pain, discomfort, and referred pain in other parts of the body. While trigger point massage is typically used to relieve muscle pain and improve posture, it can also be an effective treatment for coughing. Trigger point massage can help improve coughing by reducing tension in the muscles that control breathing. When the muscles are tense, they can put pressure on the airways, leading to coughing. Trigger point massage can help relieve this tension and improve overall respiratory function.

In addition to reducing tension in the muscles, trigger point massage can also improve circulation. Improved circulation can help the body remove irritants from the airways more effectively, reducing the likelihood of coughing. Trigger point massage can also promote relaxation, which can help reduce stress and anxiety. Stress and anxiety can lead to shallow breathing, which can increase the likelihood of coughing.

Trigger point massage is performed by applying direct pressure to the trigger points using fingers, elbows, or other tools. Your massage therapist will work with you to determine the best techniques for your individual needs. The massage may also incorporate other forms of therapy, such as aromatherapy, to help promote relaxation and improve overall health and well-being.

Massage therapy can also help to alleviate other symptoms such as headaches and fatigue that often accompany coughing. Regular massage therapy sessions can help prevent coughing from recurring by keeping the muscles and tissue in the chest and throat relaxed and healthy. Massage therapy is considered safe and effective with minimal side effects. To find a qualified massage therapist, it is important to look for a practitioner who is licensed, certified, and has received the appropriate training and education.

*Chiropractic care is* a form of alternative medicine that focuses on the diagnosis and treatment of musculoskeletal and nervous system disorders. It is based on the belief that these conditions can affect general health through the nervous system and that manual adjustment of the spine can correct these issues. While chiropractic care is primarily used to treat back and neck pain, it can also be an effective treatment for coughing.

Coughing is a common symptom of many conditions, including colds, flu, bronchitis, asthma, and even allergies. However, in some cases, coughing can be caused by problems in the musculoskeletal system, such as subluxations in the spine. These subluxations can put pressure on the nerves that control the respiratory system, leading to coughing.

Chiropractors use a variety of techniques to treat coughing, including manual adjustment of the spine, soft tissue therapy, and exercises to improve respiratory function. The goal of these treatments is to relieve pressure on the nerves that control the respiratory system and improve overall function.

Manual adjustment is the most commonly used technique for treating coughing in chiropractic care. This involves a chiropractor physically manipulating the spine to realign vertebrae and relieve pressure on the nerves. This can be done with the hands or with special tools, such as a chiropractic activator.

Soft tissue therapy is another effective treatment for coughing. This involves massaging and stretching the muscles and connective tissue around the spine to improve flexibility and reduce tension. This can help relieve pressure on the nerves and improve overall respiratory function.

Finally, chiropractors may also recommend

exercises to improve respiratory function. These can include breathing exercises, posture exercises, and physical activities that can help strengthen the muscles that control breathing.

*Tui Na* is a form of traditional Chinese massage that has been used for over 2,000 years. It is based on the principles of Chinese medicine, which views the body as a system of energy pathways (meridians) and aims to balance the flow of energy (qi) through these pathways. Tui Na involves the use of various techniques such as kneading, pressing, rubbing, and manipulating the muscles and soft tissues to improve circulation, relieve pain, and promote healing. Tui Na is often used to treat a wide range of health conditions, including coughing.

The theory behind the use of Tui Na for coughing is that the massage techniques can help to clear congestion and mucus from the lungs and improve lung function. Tui Na massage is typically applied to the back, chest, and throat area to help relieve coughing symptoms, such as tightness in the chest and throat, by relaxing the muscles and promoting breathing. This, in turn, can help to reduce coughing and improve overall respiratory function. Here is a step-by-step guide on how to perform Tui Na for coughing:

1. Find a quiet, comfortable place where you can lie down or sit comfortably. You may also want to use a pillow or cushion to support your back.

2. Begin by loosening up your neck and shoulders. Tilt your head from side to side

and roll your shoulders in a circular motion.

3. Next, focus on your chest and throat. Place your hands on your chest and gently massage the area in a circular motion, moving from the center of your chest outwards.

4. Use your fingertips to apply pressure to the points located on the side of your neck, near the top of your collarbone. Hold each point for 30 seconds.

5. Place your hands on your throat and gently massage the area in a circular motion.

6. Finally, place your hands on your abdomen and gently massage the area in a circular motion. This will help to regulate the flow of energy in your body and promote overall health.

7. Repeat the above steps for 10-15 minutes, or until you feel relaxed and relieved.

It is important to remember that Tui Na is not a substitute for medical treatment. If you have a persistent cough or any other symptoms, it is important to consult with a healthcare professional to determine the underlying cause and receive proper treatment.

## CHAPTER 14

# Homeopathy and Naturopathy for Coughing

**H**omeopathy is a form of alternative medicine that has been used for over 200 years to treat various health conditions, including coughing. Homeopathy uses highly diluted substances to stimulate the body's natural healing process. Homeopathy is based on the principle of "like cures like," meaning that a substance that causes symptoms in a healthy person can be used in small doses to treat similar symptoms in a person who is sick. While homeopathy is typically used to treat a wide range of conditions, it can also be an effective treatment for coughing. When it comes to coughing, homeopathy offers several remedies that can help relieve the symptoms. Some of the commonly used remedies include:

- **Bryonia:** This remedy is recommended for dry, hacking coughs that are accompanied by chest pain and a desire to hold the chest while coughing.

- *Drosera:* This remedy is useful for treating a persistent, spasmodic cough that worsens at night and is accompanied by a feeling of suffocation.

- *Ipecacuanha:* This remedy is indicated for

coughing that is triggered by tickling in the throat and is accompanied by nausea and vomiting.

- **Kali bichromicum:** This remedy is recommended for coughing that is caused by thick, sticky mucus that is difficult to expectorate.

- **Phosphorus:** This remedy is indicated for dry, irritating coughs that are accompanied by a feeling of tightness in the chest and a desire for cold drinks.

- **Rumex:** for a dry, tickling cough that is worse in the evening and at night.

- **Spongia:** for a dry, barking cough that is worse at night and causes difficulty breathing.

In addition to these remedies, homeopathy also offers constitutional treatment, which is tailored to the individual's unique symptoms and characteristics. This approach takes into account the person's physical, emotional, and mental symptoms, as well as their lifestyle and general health. It is important to note that homeopathic remedies are highly diluted and are safe for use in adults, children, and even pregnant women. Unlike conventional medicine, homeopathic remedies do not have any side effects and do not interact with other medications. If you are considering homeopathy for your coughing, it is best to consult with a qualified homeopathic practitioner who can recommend the appropriate remedy for your specific symptoms and needs.

*Naturopathy* is a form of alternative medicine that uses natural remedies to promote healing and prevent disease. It emphasizes the use of holistic and non-invasive treatments to help the body heal itself. When it comes to coughing, naturopathy offers several remedies that can help relieve the symptoms.

One of the main approaches used by naturopaths to treat coughing is to address the underlying cause of the cough. For example, if the cough is caused by a respiratory infection, the naturopath may recommend herbal remedies to boost the immune system and clear the infection. If the cough is caused by allergies or asthma, the naturopath may suggest dietary changes, breathing exercises, or herbal remedies to reduce inflammation and improve lung function.

Another approach used by naturopaths to treat coughing is to encourage hydration. Drinking plenty of water can help to thin mucus and make it easier to cough up. The naturopath may also recommend herbal teas, such as chamomile or marshmallow root, to soothe the throat and relieve coughing.

Naturopathic Supplements: Naturopathy often incorporates the use of supplements, such as probiotics, to support the body's natural healing processes. These supplements can help to relieve coughing by reducing inflammation and supporting the immune system.

Nutrition: Naturopathy also emphasizes the importance of proper nutrition in maintaining health and treating coughing. A diet rich in vitamins and minerals can help to strengthen the immune system and reduce coughing.

Naturopaths may also use supplements to help treat coughing. Vitamin C, for example, is a powerful antioxidant that can boost the immune system and help clear respiratory infections. Vitamin D, magnesium, and zinc are also important for maintaining respiratory health.

In addition to these remedies, naturopaths may also use breathing exercises and aromatherapy to treat coughing. Deep breathing exercises, such as diaphragmatic breathing, can help to improve lung function and reduce coughing. Aromatherapy, using essential oils such as eucalyptus or peppermint, can help to clear the airways and relieve coughing.

It is important to note that naturopathy should not be used as a substitute for conventional medical treatment. If you have a persistent cough, it is always best to see a doctor to determine the underlying cause and receive appropriate treatment.

# CHAPTER 15

# *Reflexology and Auriculotherapy for Coughing*

R*eflexology* is a form of complementary therapy that involves applying pressure to specific points on the feet, hands, or ears that are believed to correspond to specific organs and systems in the body. It is based on the idea that these reflex points can be used to stimulate healing and improve overall health and well-being. While reflexology is typically used to relieve stress and improve relaxation, it can also be an effective treatment for coughing.

Coughing is a common symptom of many conditions, including colds, flu, bronchitis, asthma, and even allergies. It is the body's natural response to remove irritants from the airways. However, in some cases, coughing can become chronic and interfere with daily life. Reflexology can help alleviate coughing by addressing the underlying causes.

Reflexology can help improve coughing by promoting relaxation and reducing stress and anxiety. When the body is relaxed and free from stress and anxiety, it is better able to remove irritants from the airways and reduce coughing. Reflexology can also stimulate the immune system, helping the body fight off infections and illnesses that can cause coughing.

- *Stimulation of the Lung Zone:* it is located on the inside of the feet, just below the ball of the foot. Stimulation of this zone can help to improve lung function and relieve coughing by increasing the flow of oxygen to the lungs and reducing inflammation.

- *Stimulation of the Sinus Zone:* it is located on the inside of the feet, near the top of the toes. Stimulation of this zone can help to relieve coughing by reducing inflammation and improving the function of the sinuses.

- *Stimulation of the Throat Zone:* it is located on the inside of the feet, near the big toe. Stimulation of this zone can help to relieve coughing and sore throat by reducing inflammation and promoting healing in the throat.

- *Stimulation of the Bronchial Tubes Zone:* it is located on the inside of the feet, near the ball of the foot. Stimulation of this zone can help to relieve coughing by reducing inflammation and improving the function of the bronchial tubes.

- *Stimulation of the Immune System Zone:* it is located on the inside of the feet, near the middle of the foot. Stimulation of this zone can help to boost the immune system and clear respiratory infections, which can reduce coughing.

- *Stimulation of the Respiratory System Zone:* it is located on the inside of the feet, near the middle of the foot. Stimulation of this zone can help to improve respiratory function and relieve coughing by reducing inflammation and increasing the flow of oxygen to the lungs.

- **Stimulation of the Chest Zone:** it is located on the inside of the feet, near the ball of the foot. Stimulation of this zone can help to relieve coughing by reducing inflammation and improving the function of the chest.

- *Stimulation of the Heart Zone:* it is located on the inside of the feet, near the big toe. Stimulation of this zone can help to relieve coughing by reducing inflammation and improving the function of the heart, which can have a positive impact on respiratory function.

- **Stimulation of the Phlegm Zone:** it is located on the inside of the feet, near the ball of the foot. Stimulation of this zone can help to relieve coughing by reducing inflammation and promoting the elimination of phlegm from the lungs.

- **Stimulation of the Allergic Reactions Zone:** it is located on the inside of the feet, near the big toe. Stimulation of this zone can help to reduce coughing and improve lung function by reducing inflammation and improving the function of the immune system.

It is important to note that these are only examples of how reflexology can treat coughing. The specific zones used and the approach used to stimulate them will depend on the individual's specific symptoms and needs.

It is best to consult with a qualified practitioner who is trained in reflexology to determine the appropriate treatment for your specific symptoms and needs.

In addition to promoting relaxation and stimulating the immune system, reflexology can also improve circulation. Improved circulation can help the body remove irritants from the airways more effectively, reducing the likelihood of coughing.

Reflexology is performed by applying pressure to specific reflex points on the feet, (even on the hands, or ears sometimes). Your reflexologist will work with you to determine the best techniques for your individual needs. The therapy may also incorporate other forms of therapy, such as aromatherapy, to help promote relaxation and improve overall health and well-being.

*Auriculotherapy,* also known as ear acupuncture, is a form of alternative medicine that uses stimulation of specific points on the ear to treat various health conditions, including coughing. It is based on the concept that the ear is a microsystem that represents the entire body. The ear has a rich network of nerves, blood vessels, and lymphatic vessels, and it is thought that stimulating specific points on the ear can affect the corresponding parts of the body. The practitioner may use needles, seed, pellets, laser or electro stimulation on the ear points to stimulate the area. Ear acupuncture can be used to treat a wide range of conditions, including respiratory issues such as coughing.

When it comes to coughing, auriculotherapy can be used to relieve the symptoms by stimulating specific points on the ear that are associated with the respiratory system. For example, stimulation of the point located near the top of the ear, which is associated with the throat, can help to relieve coughing and sore throat. Stimulation of the point located near the bottom of the ear, which is associated with the lungs, can help to improve lung function and reduce coughing. It can also be used to relieve other symptoms associated with coughing, such as chest tightness and difficulty breathing.

Auriculotherapy is typically performed using acupuncture needles, electrical stimulation, or pressure. The practitioner will first locate the specific points on the ear that correspond to the respiratory system and then apply stimulation to those points. The stimulation can be performed in a single session or several sessions, depending on the severity of the coughing and the individual's response to treatment.

- *Stimulation of the Lung Point:* The lung point is located near the bottom of the ear and is associated with the lungs. Stimulation of this point can help to improve lung function and reduce coughing by increasing the flow of oxygen to the lungs and reducing inflammation.

- *Stimulation of the Throat Point:* The throat point is located near the top of the ear and is associated with the throat. Stimulation of this point can help to relieve coughing and sore throat by reducing inflammation and promoting healing in the throat.

- *Stimulation of the Immune System Point:* The immune system point is located near the middle of the ear and is associated with the immune system. Stimulation of this point can help to boost the immune system and clear respiratory infections, which can reduce coughing.

- *Stimulation of the Bronchial Tubes Point:* The bronchial tube point is located near the bottom of the ear and is associated with the bronchial tubes. Stimulation of this point can help to relieve coughing by reducing inflammation and improving the function of the bronchial tubes.

- *Stimulation of the Respiratory System Point:* The respiratory system point is located near the middle of the ear and is associated with the respiratory system as a whole. Stimulation of this point can help to improve respiratory function and relieve coughing by reducing inflammation and increasing the flow of oxygen to the lungs.

- *Stimulation of the Sinuses Point:* The sinuses point is located near the top of the ear and is associated with the sinuses. Stimulation of this point can help to relieve coughing by reducing inflammation and improving the function of the sinuses.

- *Stimulation of the Allergic Reactions Point:* The allergic reactions point is located near the top of the ear and is associated with allergic reactions. Stimulation of this point can help to reduce coughing and improve lung function by reducing inflammation and improving the function of the immune system.

- *Stimulation of the Chest Point:* The chest point is located near the bottom of the ear and is associated with the chest. Stimulation of this point can help to relieve coughing by reducing inflammation and improving the function of the chest.

- *Stimulation of the Heart Point:* The heart point is located near the top of the ear and is associated with the heart. Stimulation of this point can help to relieve coughing by reducing inflammation and improving the function of the heart, which can have a positive impact on respiratory function.

- *Stimulation of the Phlegm Point:* The phlegm point is located near the bottom of the ear and is associated with phlegm. Stimulation of this point can help to relieve coughing by reducing inflammation and promoting the elimination of phlegm from the lungs.

It is important to note that these are only examples of how auriculotherapy can treat coughing. The specific points used and the approach used to stimulate them will depend on the individual's specific symptoms and needs. It is best to consult with a qualified practitioner who is trained in auriculotherapy to determine the appropriate treatment for your specific symptoms and needs.

*Auriculotherapy*, sometimes also referred to as *Chinese medicine ear seed therapy,* is a form of ear acupuncture that uses small seeds from the Vaccaria plant. These seeds are attached to the ear with adhesive tape and are pressed or massaged on specific points on the ear, in order to stimulate them. This therapy is based on the same principle that the ear is a microsystem that represents the entire body, and that stimulating specific points on the ear can affect the corresponding parts of the body.

In the case of coughing, ear seed therapy may be used to clear the lungs and improve lung function. It can also be used to relieve other symptoms associated with coughing, such as chest tightness and difficulty breathing. The practitioner may place the seeds on specific points on the ear that correspond to the lungs, throat, and immune system. These points are believed to help regulate the immune system, balance the energy flow in the body and help clear phlegm and mucus from the lungs.

Ear seed therapy is a non-invasive and painless method of stimulating the acupuncture points, it can be self-administered by the patient, and it is considered very safe. The seeds can be worn for several days and can be pressed or massaged by the patient at any time.

It is important to note that auriculotherapy is a safe and non-invasive form of treatment. Unlike conventional medicine, it does not have any side effects and does not interact with other medications. It can be used in combination with other treatments, such as herbal remedies or conventional medicine, to enhance the effectiveness of the treatment.

In conclusion, auriculotherapy is a safe and effective form of alternative medicine that can be used to treat coughing. By stimulating specific points on the ear that are associated with the respiratory system, auriculotherapy can help to relieve the symptoms of coughing and improve lung function. If you are considering auriculotherapy for your coughing, it is best to consult with a qualified practitioner who is trained in auriculotherapy and can recommend the appropriate treatment for your specific symptoms and needs.

# CHAPTER 16

## *Five Special Methods for Coughing*

Special methods for coughing include following:

### 1. How to stop coughing by Cupping Therapy

Cupping therapy is an ancient practice that involves the use of suction cups on the skin. The suction is created by heating the air inside the cup, which causes a vacuum to form when the cup is placed on the skin. The suction created by the cups is thought to help increase blood flow, reduce inflammation, and relieve pain. Cupping therapy has been used for centuries in traditional Chinese medicine and is believed to be beneficial for a wide range of conditions. It is commonly used to treat musculoskeletal conditions such as back and neck pain, but it has also been used to treat respiratory conditions such as asthma and chronic bronchitis.

Cupping therapy is thought to help relieve coughing by increasing blood flow to the lungs and helping to clear mucus from the airways. This therapy is often used in combination with other traditional Chinese medicine techniques such as acupuncture and herbal medicine to help relieve coughing. There is some evidence to suggest that cupping therapy may be effective in reducing coughing. A systematic review and meta-analysis of randomized controlled trials published in the Journal of Traditional Chinese Medicine found that cupping therapy may be effective in reducing coughing caused by respiratory conditions such as chronic bronchitis and asthma.

Cupping therapy is generally considered safe when performed by a trained practitioner, but it can cause skin irritation and bruising. It's important to speak with a healthcare professional before trying cupping therapy, especially if you have a

## 2. How to stop coughing by Gua Sha Scraping

Gua sha is a traditional Chinese healing technique that involves scraping the skin with a smooth-edged tool to stimulate blood flow and reduce muscle tension. Gua sha has been traditionally used to treat a wide range of health conditions, including coughing. The theory behind the use of gua sha for coughing is that the scraping motion of the tool can help to break up congestion and clear mucus from the lungs, thus reducing coughing. Gua sha scraping is typically performed on the back, chest, and throat area to help open up the airways and relieve coughing symptoms.

Gua sha is a technique that should be performed by a qualified practitioner, who can properly guide and supervise it, to avoid any injury or adverse effects. It's also important to mention that gua sha scraping can cause skin irritation and bruising, so it's important to talk to a qualified practitioner before trying it, to make sure that you are a good candidate for this technique. Gua sha is not suitable for everyone, and some people should avoid it altogether. It's not recommended for those with sensitive skin, eczema, psoriasis, or active skin infections. It's also not recommended for people who are on blood thinners or have blood clotting disorders.

Although gua sha may be helpful for certain symptoms, it's not suitable for everyone, and it is not a substitute for conventional medical treatment. If you have a persistent cough, it's important to consult with a healthcare professional to determine the underlying cause and to receive proper treatment.

### 3. How to stop coughing by Moxibustion

Moxibustion is a traditional Chinese healing technique that involves the burning of the herb mugwort, or moxa, on or near the skin in order to stimulate healing and improve circulation. It is often used in conjunction with acupuncture to treat a wide range of health conditions, including coughing. The theory behind the use of moxibustion for coughing is that the heat generated by the burning moxa can help to open up the airways and clear mucus from the lungs. Moxibustion is typically applied to acupuncture points on the back, chest, and throat to help relieve coughing symptoms.

There is some evidence to suggest that moxibustion may be effective in treating coughing caused by respiratory conditions such as asthma and bronchitis. A study published in the Journal of Traditional Chinese Medicine found that moxibustion improved lung function and reduced coughing in patients with chronic obstructive pulmonary disease.

It's important to note that while moxibustion may be helpful for certain symptoms, it should not be used as a substitute for conventional medical treatment. It's always best to consult with a healthcare professional before trying moxibustion or any other alternative therapy, and it's also important to have a qualified practitioner to guide and supervise the practice.

## *4. How to stop coughing by CBD Oil*

CBD oil, also known as cannabidiol, is a compound found in the cannabis plant. It is believed to work by interacting with the body's endocannabinoid system, which is a system of receptors that play a role in regulating various physiological processes, including pain, mood, and inflammation. There is some research that suggests that CBD oil may have potential as a treatment for coughing. A study published in the European Journal of Pain found that CBD oil may help reduce coughing caused by chronic obstructive pulmonary disease (COPD).

CBD oil is available in different forms, such as tinctures, capsules, gummies, topicals and vapes. The most common method of use is through oral consumption of CBD oil in the form of tinctures or capsules. When it comes to using CBD oil for coughing, it's important to note that there is limited research on its effects. While some studies suggest that CBD oil may be effective in reducing coughing caused by conditions such as COPD and asthma, more research is needed to confirm these findings. Another study published in the Journal of Clinical Psychology found that CBD oil may help reduce coughing caused by asthma. However, it's important to note that more research is needed to understand the full effects of CBD oil on coughing, and it's not clear what dosage or form of CBD oil would be most effective.

It's also important to mention that CBD products are not yet regulated by the FDA, so it's difficult to know exactly what you're getting when you purchase them. It's important to speak with a healthcare professional before taking any new supplement or medication, including CBD oil, especially if you're taking other medications. It's also important to note that CBD oil may have side effects, such as drowsiness, changes in appetite, and changes in weight. CBD oil may also interact with certain medications, so it's important to speak with a professional before taking it if you're taking other medications. It is also worth mentioning that CBD is derived from hemp and marijuana, hemp-derived CBD is legal in many countries while marijuana-derived CBD is illegal in most countries. So, it's important to check the laws and regulations of your country before using CBD oil.

In summary, while there is some research suggesting that CBD oil may be effective in reducing coughing, more research is needed to confirm these findings. It's important to speak with a healthcare professional before taking CBD oil, especially if you're taking other medications.

## 5. How to stop coughing by Chakra Energy System

The chakra energy system is a concept found in ancient Indian and Hindu traditions, which describes seven energy centers in the body, each associated with a specific area of the physical and emotional body. Each chakra is thought to be responsible for a different aspect of physical and emotional health, and when they are blocked or out of balance, it can lead to various health problems, including coughing.

The chakra associated with the lungs and the throat is the fifth chakra, known as the Vishuddha chakra. This chakra is located at the base of the neck and is associated with communication, self-expression, and the ability to release emotions. According to the chakra system, coughing can be caused by blockages in the Vishuddha chakra. The blockages can manifest physically as a tightness in the throat, difficulty breathing, or a persistent cough. Some techniques that can be used to balance the Vishuddha chakra include:

Chanting: Chanting mantras or affirmations associated with the Vishuddha chakra can help to unblock and balance the energy in this chakra.

Yoga: Certain yoga poses, such as the Fish pose or the Camel pose, can help to open and balance the Vishuddha chakra.

Meditation: Meditating on the color of the Vishuddha chakra, which is blue, can help to balance the energy in this chakra.

Singing: Singing or humming can help to open the throat chakra and release any blockages.

If you are considering incorporating chakra

balancing techniques into your healthcare routine, it's important to speak with a qualified practitioner who can guide you through the process and ensure that the techniques you are using are safe and appropriate for your individual needs. The chakra energy system is an ancient concept found in Indian and Hindu traditions, it's not recognized as a valid form of treatment by modern medicine, and scientific research has not yet confirmed its effectiveness. While certain techniques such as yoga, meditation, and chanting can be beneficial for overall health and well-being, they should not be used as a substitute for conventional medical treatment for chronic coughing.

If you have a persistent cough, it's essential to consult with a healthcare professional to determine the underlying cause of the coughing.

# CHAPTER 17

## *Ancient Medicines for Coughing*

*H*ow did ancient Indian *people treat coughing?*

**Ayurveda** is an ancient Indian medicine that has been practiced in India for over 5,000 years. It is based on the belief that good health is achieved by maintaining a balance between the mind, body, and spirit. Ayurveda classifies individuals into three doshas: vata, pitta, and kapha, which correspond to different physical and mental characteristics.

Ayurveda views coughing because of an imbalance in the body's doshas. According to Ayurveda, coughing can be caused by a variety of factors, including an excess of kapha, which can lead to congested respiratory passages, or an imbalance of vata and pitta, which can lead to dryness and irritation in the throat. Ayurvedic remedies aim to restore balance to the body and address the underlying cause of coughing. These remedies may include dietary changes, herbal remedies, and lifestyle modifications. Here is a step-by-step guide on how to use Ayurveda to stop coughing. Identify your dosha type. This can be done through an Ayurvedic consultation with a practitioner or by taking an online quiz.

1. Make dietary changes to balance your dosha: Ayurvedic practitioners may recommend changes to

diet and lifestyle to help balance the body and reduce the symptoms of coughing. For example, they may recommend avoiding foods that are considered to be aggravating to the condition, such as cold or spicy foods. Or if you have an excess of kapha, you may want to reduce heavy, oily, and sweet foods, and instead focus on lighter foods.

2. Herbal remedies: Ayurvedic practitioners may recommend herbal formulations such as licorice root, ginger, turmeric, and licorice root, which are believed to have anti-inflammatory and expectorant properties that can help to soothe the throat and clear mucus from the lungs, which can help to reduce coughing.

3. Panchakarma: Panchakarma is a type of Ayurvedic detoxification treatment that is believed to help balance the body and reduce the symptoms of coughing. It includes a series of therapeutic procedures such as massage, herbal steam baths, and enemas.

4. Yoga and breathing exercises: Ayurvedic practitioners may also recommend yoga and breathing exercises to help balance the body and reduce the symptoms of coughing. It is important to practice stress-management techniques, such as meditation and yoga, to help calm the mind and body. These exercises are believed to help improve lung function and promote deep breathing, which can help to clear mucus from the lungs.

5. Use aromatherapy: Essential oils such as eucalyptus, peppermint, and thyme can be used in a diffuser or added to a steam bath to help clear congested respiratory passages.

It is important to remember that Ayurveda is not a substitute for medical treatment. If you have a persistent cough or any other symptoms, it is important to consult with a healthcare professional to determine the underlying cause and receive proper treatment. Seek the advice of an Ayurvedic practitioner. An Ayurvedic practitioner can provide personalized recommendations based on your individual needs and health history.

## How did ancient Greek people treat coughing?

Ancient Greeks had a developed understanding of medicine and used various methods to treat coughing. They inherited a lot of knowledge from the Greek civilization. They used both herbal remedies and surgical procedures to treat coughing. The ancient Greeks believed that coughing was caused by an imbalance in the body's humors (blood, phlegm, yellow bile, and black bile) and treated it with a combination of herbal remedies and dietary changes.

Herbal remedies were commonly used to treat coughing, and the ancient Romans had a wide variety of plants and herbs at their disposal. Some of the plants that were used include thyme, which was believed to have expectorant properties, and hyssop, which was used to treat respiratory conditions. They also used licorice root and marshmallow root as a remedy for coughing. The use of honey and poppy was also popular as a remedy for coughing.

Ancient Greek physicians such as Hippocrates,

Galen, and Dioscorides wrote extensively on the treatment of coughing. They recommended treatments such as inhaling steam infused with herbs, drinking warm liquids, and using expectorants to help clear mucus from the lungs.

Surgeons in ancient Greece were also highly skilled and performed a wide range of surgical procedures to treat coughing. These procedures included the removal of polyps or tumors in the nose and throat, which could cause coughing, as well as the surgical repair of the trachea or bronchi to relieve coughing.

In addition to these remedies, the ancient Romans also believed in the power of magic and religion to heal. They performed religious rituals, spells and incantations to treat coughing. They also used amulets and charms to protect the person from the evil spirits believed to cause the coughing.

It's worth noting that these ancient remedies have not been scientifically proven to be effective in stopping coughs and some of them may even be dangerous, so it's always best to consult with a doctor before trying any home remedies.

## How did ancient Egypt people treat coughing?

Ancient Egyptians had a sophisticated understanding of medicine and used various methods to treat coughing. They had a wide variety of remedies and treatments which included both herbal remedies and surgical procedures.

Herbal remedies were commonly used to treat coughing, with a wide range of plants and herbs being used for this purpose. Some of the plants that were used include thyme, which was believed to have expectorant properties, and frankincense, which was used to treat respiratory conditions. The ancient Egyptians used a variety of remedies to treat coughing, including honey, garlic, and myrrh.

Surgeons in ancient Egypt were highly skilled and performed a wide range of surgical procedures to treat coughing. These procedures included the removal of polyps or tumors in the nose and throat, which could cause coughing, as well as the surgical repair of the trachea or bronchi to relieve coughing.

In addition to these remedies, the ancient Egyptians also believed in the power of magic and religion to heal. They performed religious rituals, spells and incantations to treat coughing. They also used amulets and charms to protect the person from the evil spirits believed to cause the coughing.

It's worth noting that these ancient remedies have not been scientifically proven to be effective in stopping coughs and some of them may even be dangerous, so it's always best to consult with a doctor before trying any home remedies.

## How did ancient African people treat coughing

Traditional African medicine, also known as indigenous African medicine, is a diverse set of practices used by different ethnic groups across Africa to prevent, diagnose and treat illnesses. The specific treatment for coughing may vary depending on the specific ethnic group, but generally traditional African medicine relies heavily on the use of plants and herbs for medicinal purposes.

Herbal remedies were commonly used to treat coughing, and many different plants and herbs were used for this purpose. Some examples of plants that were used include:

Aframomum melegueta (alligator pepper) which is believed to have expectorant and antimicrobial properties, was used to treat coughs and chest infections.

Hyptis suaveolens (pignut) was used to treat respiratory conditions and coughing

Zingiber officinale (ginger) is believed to have anti-inflammatory properties that can help to soothe the throat and suppress coughing.

In addition to herbal remedies, traditional African medicine also includes other methods such as spiritual and supernatural practices, rituals and ceremonies. Some ethnic groups may also use traditional healers, known as "sangomas" or "witch doctors" to perform rituals and incantations to treat coughing.

It's worth noting that these traditional remedies have not been scientifically proven to be effective in stopping coughs and some of them may even be dangerous, so it's always best to consult with a doctor before trying any home remedies.

# CHAPTER 18

# *Prescription Medications for Severe Coughing*

S evere coughing can be a debilitating and disruptive symptom that can impact your daily life. While over-the-counter (OTC) medications can be effective for mild to moderate coughing, severe coughing may require prescription medications.

### Antibiotics

Some severe and persistent coughing should be a bacterial infection, and antibiotics may be prescribed to help treat the infection and relieve the symptoms of coughing. Antibiotics are medications that work by killing or inhibiting the growth of bacteria that cause infections. They are specifically designed to target bacteria and are not effective against viruses, which are a common cause of respiratory infections. Antibiotics are classified into different groups, including *penicillin, cephalosporins, macrolides, and fluoroquinolones*. The specific antibiotic used to treat severe coughing will depend on the underlying condition and the type of bacteria causing the infection.

Common Antibiotics for Respiratory Infections: *amoxicillin, azithromycin, and clarithromycin.* These medications are available in different forms, including oral tablets and liquids, and intravenous injections. The specific antibiotic used to treat severe coughing will depend on the underlying condition and the severity of symptoms. The recommended dose and administration of antibiotics will vary depending on the specific medication and the underlying condition being treated. It is essential to follow the recommended dosage and administration instructions provided by your doctor or pharmacist. Antibiotics should be taken as directed and should not be stopped early, even if symptoms improve. This can increase the risk of antibiotic resistance and make it more difficult to treat future infections.

It is important to consult a doctor before taking antibiotics for severe coughing. Your doctor will perform a thorough evaluation to determine the underlying cause of your coughing and recommend the best course of treatment. Antibiotics are not recommended for individuals with a history of allergies or sensitivity to antibiotics, as they can cause adverse effects. It is also important to inform your doctor if you are pregnant, breastfeeding, or taking other medications, as antibiotics can interact with some medications and cause adverse effects. Antibiotics should only be used to treat bacterial infections and should not be used to treat viral infections, as they are not effective against viruses.

### Mucolytics

Mucolytics are a class of prescription medications that work by thinning mucus, making it easier to cough up. These medications are often used to treat conditions such as bronchitis, chronic obstructive pulmonary disease (COPD), and cystic fibrosis. Mucolytics work by breaking down the bonds between the mucus molecules, making the mucus thinner and easier to cough up. This helps to clear the airways of mucus and other irritants, reducing coughing and making it easier to breathe. Mucolytics also help to keep the mucus from becoming too thick, which can make it harder to cough up and lead to further respiratory problems.

### Common Mucolytics

*Acetylcysteine (AC):* AC is available in oral and intravenous formulations and is often used to treat respiratory conditions such as bronchitis, COPD, and cystic fibrosis. *Carbocisteine* is available in oral and topical formulations and is often used to treat respiratory conditions such as bronchitis, COPD, and pharyngitis.

The recommended dose and administration of mucolytics will vary depending on the specific medication and the underlying condition being treated. It is essential to follow the recommended dosage and administration instructions provided by your doctor or pharmacist. Overdosing on mucolytics can lead to serious adverse effects, including bronchospasm, nausea, and vomiting. It is important to consult a doctor before taking mucolytics for severe coughing. Your doctor will perform a thorough evaluation to determine the underlying cause of your coughing and recommend the best course of treatment. Mucolytics are not recommended for individuals with a history of bronchospasm or other respiratory conditions. It is also important to inform your doctor if you are pregnant, breastfeeding, or taking other medications, as mucolytics can interact with some medications and cause adverse effects.

### Bronchodilators

Bronchodilators are a class of prescription medications that work by relaxing the smooth muscles in the airways, making it easier to breathe and reducing coughing. These medications are often used to treat conditions such as asthma, chronic obstructive pulmonary disease (COPD), and bronchitis. Bronchodilators work by relaxing the smooth muscles in the airways, making it easier to breathe and reducing coughing. This helps to clear the airways of mucus and other irritants, reducing coughing and making it easier to breathe. Bronchodilators also help to keep the airways open, which can prevent further respiratory problems.

Some of the most commonly used bronchodilators include *albuterol, levalbuterol, salmeterol, and formoterol.* Albuterol is a short-acting bronchodilator that is often used to treat acute asthma symptoms. Salmeterol and formoterol are long-acting bronchodilators that are often used to control the symptoms of asthma and COPD.

The recommended dose and administration of bronchodilators will vary depending on the specific medication and the underlying condition being treated. It is essential to follow the recommended dosage and administration instructions provided by your doctor or pharmacist. Overdosing on bronchodilators can lead to serious adverse effects, including rapid heart rate, tremor, and nervousness. Bronchodilators are not recommended for individuals with a history of heart problems or other serious medical conditions. It is also important to inform your doctor if you are pregnant, breastfeeding, or taking other medications, as bronchodilators can interact with some medications and cause adverse effects.

### Steroids

Steroids may be prescribed to help reduce the severity of coughing. Steroids are a class of medications that work by reducing inflammation in the body, which can help to relieve symptoms associated with respiratory conditions. Steroids work by reducing inflammation in the body. This helps to relieve symptoms associated with respiratory conditions such as bronchitis, asthma, and chronic obstructive pulmonary disease (COPD). Steroids also help to reduce the production of mucus, which can help to clear the airways and reduce coughing.

Common Steroids: *prednisone, dexamethasone, and methylprednisolone.* These medications are available in different forms, including oral tablets, inhalers, and injectables. The specific steroid used to treat severe coughing will depend on the underlying condition and the severity of symptoms. The recommended dose and administration of steroids will vary depending on the specific medication and the underlying condition being treated. It is essential to follow the recommended dosage and administration instructions provided by your doctor or pharmacist. Overdosing on steroids can lead to serious adverse effects, including weight gain, mood changes, and decreased immunity.

Steroid Inhalers, also known as corticosteroid

inhalers, such as **Fluticasone**. They are commonly used to treat conditions such as asthma and chronic obstructive pulmonary disease (COPD). Fluticasone is a common steroid inhaler that is available by prescription. Fluticasone works by reducing the inflammation in the airways that can cause symptoms such as coughing, wheezing, and shortness of breath. It is inhaled directly into the lungs, where it works to reduce inflammation and open up the airways.

It's important to note that steroid inhalers are not a cure for conditions such as asthma or COPD, they only help to relieve the symptoms. People with these conditions should consult with their healthcare provider for a proper treatment plan. Additionally, people with certain medical conditions such as osteoporosis, diabetes, or heart disease should consult with their healthcare provider before taking steroid inhalers as they may not be suitable for them. It's also important to follow the instructions on the package or as advised by the healthcare professional and not to exceed the recommended dosage. Long-term use of steroid inhalers can lead to side effects such as oral thrush, hoarseness, and even decreased bone density, so it's important to use them as directed by a healthcare professional.

It is important to consult a doctor before taking steroids for severe coughing. Your doctor will perform a thorough evaluation to determine the underlying cause of your coughing and recommend the best course of treatment. Steroids are not recommended for individuals with a history of heart problems or other serious medical conditions. It is also important to inform your doctor if you are pregnant, breastfeeding, or taking other medications, as steroids can interact with some medications and cause adverse effects.

### Antitussives

Cough suppressants, also known as antitussives, are medications that work by reducing the reflex that causes coughing. They are used to relieve the symptoms of a cough, rather than treating the underlying cause. Antitussives could be prescribed to help relieve the symptoms of coughing. Antitussives are a class of medications that work by suppressing the cough reflex and reducing the frequency and severity of coughing. Antitussives work by suppressing the cough reflex in the brain. This helps to reduce the frequency and severity of coughing. Antitussives are generally classified into two categories: centrally-acting and peripherally-acting. Centrally-acting antitussives work by suppressing the cough reflex in the brain, while peripherally-acting antitussives work by reducing the sensitivity of the cough receptors in the airways.

Common Antitussives: ***dextromethorphan, codeine, and benzonatate***. These medications are available in different forms, including oral syrups, tablets, and lozenges. The specific antitussive used to treat severe coughing will depend on the underlying condition and the severity of symptoms. The recommended dose and administration of antitussives will vary depending on the specific medication and the underlying condition being treated. It is essential to follow the recommended dosage and administration instructions provided by your doctor or pharmacist. Overdosing on antitussives can lead to serious adverse effects, including drowsiness, confusion, and difficulty breathing.

**Dextromethorphan** is the most commonly used cough suppressant. It is available over-the-counter in liquid and pill form, and it works by reducing the activity of the cough center in the brain. It is considered safe for most people, but it can cause side effects such as drowsiness, dizziness, and nausea, and can interact with other medications.

**Codeine** is a medication that is used as a cough suppressant and pain reliever. It is an opioid medication, which means it works by binding to specific receptors in the brain and spinal cord to reduce pain and suppress coughing. Codeine is typically administered in the form of a tablet or liquid. The tablet form is taken by mouth, and the liquid form is usually taken by mouth or through an oral syringe. It's usually taken every 4 to 6 hours as needed for pain or coughing. Codeine is usually prescribed in combination with other medications to provide more effective relief. For example, it's often combined with antihistamines or decongestants for relief of coughing.

Codeine is considered a controlled substance by the U.S. Food and Drug Administration (FDA) due to its potential for addiction, abuse and overdose. And it can have side effects like drowsiness, dizziness, nausea, and constipation. Codeine can also interact with other medications, so it's important to consult with a doctor before taking it, especially if you're already taking other medications. And it's not recommended for long-term use, and should be used only as directed by your doctor. Additionally, Codeine can cause severe respiratory depression if taken in high doses or when combined with other CNS depressants, such as alcohol or other sedative/hypnotic drugs, which can be fatal. And tolerance, physical and psychological dependence can occur with prolonged use, which can lead to addiction.

It is important to note that cough suppressants should not be used to treat a cough that is caused by a serious underlying condition, such as pneumonia, bronchitis, or asthma. And as with any medication, it's always recommended to consult with your doctor before taking a cough suppressant, and to follow the recommended dosage and usage instructions. Additionally, it's important to be aware of the potential side effects and to consult with your doctor if you have any concerns or experience any side effects. Cough suppressants are not recommended for children under 4 years old, and it's not recommended for coughs caused by smoking, emphysema, or asthma.

It is important to consult a doctor before taking antitussives for severe coughing. Your doctor will perform a thorough evaluation to determine the underlying cause of your coughing and recommend the best course of treatment. Antitussives are not recommended for individuals with a history of liver or kidney problems, as they can be metabolized and eliminated from the body through these organs. It is also important to inform your doctor if you are pregnant, breastfeeding, or taking other medications, as antitussives can interact with some medications and cause adverse effects.

### Antihistamines

Antihistamines are medications that block the

effects of histamine, a chemical produced by the body in response to an allergen. Histamine causes inflammation, swelling, and irritation in the airways, which can lead to coughing. By blocking histamine, antihistamines can help reduce coughing, sneezing, and other symptoms of allergies. Choose the right antihistamine: There are many different types of antihistamines, including first-generation and second-generation. First-generation antihistamines are older medications that can cause drowsiness, while second-generation antihistamines are newer and less likely to cause drowsiness. Your doctor will recommend the best type of antihistamine for your condition based on your individual needs.

First-generation antihistamines are also known as sedating antihistamines, because they can cause drowsiness as a side effect. They include medications such as *diphenhydramine (Benadryl) and chlorpheniramine (Chlor-Trimeton)*. These antihistamines are effective in relieving symptoms such as sneezing and a runny nose, but they can cause drowsiness and impair cognitive function, which is why they are usually recommended for use at bedtime.

Second-generation antihistamines, also known as non-sedating antihistamines, have less sedative effects, and they include medications such as *cetirizine (Zyrtec), fexofenadine (Allegra), and loratadine (Claritin)*. These antihistamines are less likely to cause drowsiness and cognitive impairment, making them a better option for use during the day.

*Loratadine* is a second-generation antihistamine that works by blocking the effects of histamine, a substance that causes coughing, runny nose, and watery eyes. It is available in tablet form and can be found in several allergy medications such as Claritin and Alavert. Loratadine is considered safe for most people and does not cause drowsiness, making it an excellent option for individuals who cannot tolerate drowsiness caused by some antihistamines.

*Cetirizine* is another second-generation antihistamine that works by blocking the effects of histamine. It is available in tablet form and can be found in several allergy medications such as Zyrtec and Reactine. Cetirizine is considered safe for most people and does not cause drowsiness, making it an excellent option for individuals who cannot tolerate drowsiness caused by some antihistamines.

*Fexofenadine* is a second-generation antihistamine that is available by prescription. It is effective in reducing the symptoms of allergies, including coughing. Fexofenadine works by blocking histamine receptors, reducing inflammation and irritation in the airways. It is less likely to cause drowsiness compared to first-generation antihistamines, making it a good choice for those who need to stay alert during the day.

Follow the instructions carefully: When taking antihistamines, it is important to follow the instructions carefully. This includes the recommended dose, frequency, and duration of use. Overuse of antihistamines can lead to adverse side effects, such as drowsiness, dizziness, and blurred vision. Take antihistamines at the right time: For maximum effectiveness, antihistamines should be taken at the right time. If your coughing is worse at night, for example, it is best to take the antihistamine before bed. Your doctor will advise you on the best time to take your antihistamines based on your individual needs.

### Other Treatments for Severe Coughing:

- *Oxygen therapy:* Oxygen therapy is a medical procedure that involves the delivery of oxygen to the lungs to help improve breathing. It is commonly used to treat conditions such as COPD and cystic fibrosis. Oxygen therapy can be administered through a nasal cannula or mask.

- *Pulmonary rehabilitation:* Pulmonary rehabilitation is a medical program that involves a combination of exercise, education, and support for individuals with lung disease. It can help to reduce coughing and improve overall lung function.

- *Lung surgery:* Lung surgery is a medical procedure that involves the removal of a portion of the lung to treat conditions such as lung cancer and emphysema. It can help to reduce coughing and improve overall lung function.

- *Pleural effusion drainage:* Pleural effusion drainage is a medical procedure that involves the removal of excess fluid that has built up in the pleural cavity, which can cause coughing. It is commonly used to treat conditions such as pneumonia and lung cancer.

- *Tracheostomy:* Tracheostomy is a medical procedure that involves the creation of an opening in the neck through which a tube is inserted into the trachea to help with breathing. It is commonly used to treat conditions such as COPD and sleep apnea.

- ***Extracorporeal membrane oxygenation (ECMO):*** Extracorporeal membrane oxygenation (ECMO) is a medical procedure that uses a machine to oxygenate the blood outside the body. It is commonly used to treat severe respiratory failure, and it can help to reduce coughing and improve overall lung function.

# CHAPTER 19

## *Coughing Due To Sixteen Different Diseases*

*oughing due to Influenza:*

**C** Coughing is a common symptom of many respiratory conditions, including the flu. The flu, or influenza, is a viral infection that affects the respiratory system and can cause symptoms such as fever, fatigue, body aches, and a persistent cough. Understanding the connection between coughing and the flu can help you better manage your symptoms and make informed decisions about your health.

The flu can cause a persistent cough for several reasons. First, the virus can cause inflammation in the airways, leading to coughing. Second, the flu can also cause excess mucus production, which can lead to coughing as the body tries to clear the airways. Third, coughing is a natural reflex that helps the body clear mucus, bacteria, and other irritants from the respiratory system. In the case of the flu, coughing can help the body clear the virus and prevent further spread of the infection.

It is important to distinguish between a persistent cough due to the flu and other causes of coughing, such as allergies, sinusitis, or pneumonia. A cough due to the flu will typically resolve within a week or two and may be accompanied by other flu symptoms, such as fever, fatigue, and body aches. If your cough persists longer than two weeks or is accompanied by other symptoms, such as chest pain or shortness of breath, it is important to see your doctor for further evaluation.

Treatment for a persistent cough due to the flu typically involves managing the symptoms and supporting the body's natural healing process. This may include rest, hydration, over-the-counter pain relievers, and decongestants. In some cases, antiviral medications may be prescribed to shorten the duration of the flu and reduce the risk of complications.

In addition to these measures, there are several things you can do to help manage your cough and prevent the spread of the flu:

- Cover your mouth and nose when coughing or sneezing: Covering your mouth and nose with a tissue or the inside of your elbow can help prevent the spread of the flu to others.

- Wash your hands frequently: Wash your hands frequently with soap and water for at least 20 seconds to help prevent the spread of germs.

- Avoid close contact with others: Stay home and avoid close contact with others until your symptoms have resolved. This can help prevent the spread of the flu to others.

- Get vaccinated: The flu vaccine is the best way to prevent the flu and reduce the risk of complications. The vaccine is recommended for everyone over the age of 6 months, especially those at high risk for complications, such as people with underlying medical conditions and older adults.

### Coughing due to Asthma

Coughing is a common symptom of asthma, a chronic respiratory condition that affects millions of people worldwide. Asthma is characterized by inflammation and narrowing of the airways, which can make breathing difficult and lead to persistent coughing. Understanding the connection between coughing and asthma can help you better manage your symptoms and prevent exacerbations.

Asthma is a complex condition that affects the airways, causing them to become inflamed and narrow. This narrowing can cause symptoms such as wheezing, shortness of breath, chest tightness, and a persistent cough. In some cases, the cough may be the only symptom of asthma. The cough can be dry or productive and may be worse at night, in the morning, or after exercise. There are several factors that can trigger an asthma exacerbation, including exposure to allergens, viral infections, air pollution, and physical activity. It is important to identify your personal triggers and take steps to avoid them in order to prevent exacerbations.

Diagnosis of asthma is typically based on a combination of medical history, physical examination, and diagnostic tests, such as spirometry and skin prick tests. Once a diagnosis of asthma is made, your doctor will work with you to develop a management plan that includes lifestyle modifications, medications, and regular follow-up visits.

Treatment for asthma typically involves a combination of medications and lifestyle modifications.

- Medications: Cough-variant asthma is managed with medications such as bronchodilators and inhaled corticosteroids to help open up the airways and reduce inflammation, making it easier to cough up mucus. Long-acting bronchodilators, such as salmeterol, are commonly used to help control symptoms. Inhaled corticosteroids are also commonly used to prevent exacerbations and reduce inflammation in the airways.

There are two main types of medications used to treat asthma: quick-relief medications and long-term control medications. Quick-relief medications are used to provide immediate relief from symptoms during an asthma attack. Long-term control medications are used to prevent symptoms and reduce the frequency and severity of asthma attacks. Some common medications used to treat asthma include:

1. Quick-relief medications:
- Short-acting beta agonists (SABAs)
- Anticholinergics

2. Long-term control medications:

- Inhaled corticosteroids
- Leukotriene modifiers
- Long-acting beta agonists (LABAs)
- Theophylline

- Inhalers: Inhalers are devices that deliver medication directly to the lungs and are commonly used to manage cough-variant asthma. They come in different forms, such as metered-dose inhalers, dry powder inhalers, and nebulizers.
- Avoiding triggers: Identifying and avoiding triggers that can cause coughing, such as smoke, dust, pollen, and chemical fumes, is an important aspect of managing cough-variant asthma.
- Pulmonary rehabilitation: Pulmonary rehabilitation is a program that includes exercise, education, and support for individuals with lung disease. It can help to improve lung function and reduce coughing in people with cough variant asthma.
- Monitoring symptoms: Regularly monitoring symptoms, such as coughing, shortness of breath, and chest tightness, is an important aspect of managing cough-variant asthma. Keeping a symptom diary can help individuals and healthcare providers identify triggers and track the effectiveness of treatment.
- Action plan: Having an action plan in place, developed in collaboration with

a healthcare provider, is important for managing cough-variant asthma. The plan should include information on how to recognize symptoms, how to respond to exacerbations, and when to seek medical attention.

- Educating oneself: Educating oneself about the condition and its management is important for managing cough-variant asthma. Understanding the disease, its triggers, and treatment options can help individuals to better manage their condition and reduce coughing.
- Support groups: Joining a support group for individuals with asthma can provide emotional and social support, as well as access to information and resources that can help to manage coughing associated with this condition.
- Allergen immunotherapy: Allergen immunotherapy, also known as allergy shots, can help to reduce coughing by reducing the body's sensitivity to allergens. It involves receiving injections of allergens over a period of time to help the body become less sensitive to them.
- Nasal irrigation: Nasal irrigation is a technique that involves flushing the nasal passages with a saline solution to help clear mucus and reduce inflammation. It can be helpful in managing cough-variant asthma, as it can help to reduce nasal congestion and coughing.

- Steam therapy: Steam therapy can help to reduce coughing by loosening mucus and reducing inflammation in the nasal passages and sinuses. It can be done by taking a hot shower or using a humidifier.
- Oxygen therapy: In some cases, oxygen therapy may be used to help manage cough-variant asthma, especially in people who have low oxygen levels in the blood. It involves the delivery of oxygen to the lungs, which can help to reduce coughing and improve breathing.

### *Coughing due to Bronchitis*

Bronchitis is a respiratory condition that is characterized by inflammation of the bronchial tubes, the airways that carry air to and from the lungs. Coughing is a common symptom of bronchitis, and can range from a mild, occasional cough to a persistent, debilitating cough. Understanding the connection between coughing and bronchitis can help you better manage your symptoms and prevent complications. Bronchitis can be caused by a variety of factors, including viral infections, exposure to air pollution, and cigarette smoke. The condition can be acute, meaning it develops suddenly and lasts for a short period of time, or chronic, meaning it develops over time and persists for several months or even years.

Acute bronchitis is typically caused by a viral infection, such as the common cold or flu. Symptoms can include a persistent cough, wheezing, shortness of breath, and chest tightness. The cough is usually productive, meaning it produces mucus, and can last for several weeks.

Chronic bronchitis, on the other hand, is a type of chronic obstructive pulmonary disease (COPD) that is typically caused by long-term exposure to irritants, such as cigarette smoke or air pollution. Symptoms can include a persistent cough that produces mucus, wheezing, shortness of breath, and chest tightness.

Diagnosis of bronchitis is typically based on a combination of medical history, physical examination, and diagnostic tests, such as spirometry and chest X-rays. Once a diagnosis of bronchitis is made, your doctor will work with you to develop a management plan that includes lifestyle modifications, medications, and regular follow-up visits.

Treatment for bronchitis typically involves a combination of medications and lifestyle modifications. Medications used to treat bronchitis include bronchodilators, which can help relieve symptoms by opening up the airways, and expectorants, which can help to reduce mucus production and improve cough symptoms. Lifestyle modifications may include avoiding triggers, such as cigarette smoke and air pollution, and engaging in regular physical activity.

In addition to these measures, there are several things you can do to help manage your symptoms and prevent complications:

- Take your medications as prescribed: Follow your doctor's instructions for taking your medications, including the correct dosing and frequency.

- Avoid triggers: Identify your personal triggers and take steps to avoid them in order to prevent exacerbations.

- Practice good respiratory hygiene: Cover your mouth and nose when coughing or sneezing and wash your hands frequently to prevent the spread of germs.

- Monitor your symptoms: Keep track of your symptoms, including the frequency and severity of your coughing, and share this information with your doctor.

- Get vaccinated: Get vaccinated against common respiratory infections, such as the flu, to help prevent exacerbations of bronchitis

### *Coughing due to Sinusitis:*

Sinusitis, also known as sinus infection, is a common condition that can lead to a persistent cough. It occurs when the sinuses, which are the cavities in the skull that produce mucus, become inflamed and congested. This can lead to a range of symptoms, including nasal congestion, headache, and a persistent cough. The cause of sinusitis can be due to a variety of factors, including a viral or bacterial infection, structural abnormalities in the sinuses, or an underlying condition, such as allergies or asthma. In some cases, sinusitis can also be caused by environmental factors, such as exposure to pollution or changes in the weather.

Diagnosis of sinusitis typically begins with a thorough medical history and physical examination. Your doctor may also recommend additional diagnostic tests, such as a CT scan or an x-ray, to confirm the diagnosis and determine the extent of the infection.

Treatment for sinusitis typically involves managing the underlying cause of the condition. In many cases, this may involve antibiotics or other medications to reduce inflammation and relieve symptoms.

1.   Other Medications: Sinusitis are managed with medications such as antihistamines, decongestants, and corticosteroids to help reduce inflammation and relieve symptoms such as coughing. Antihistamines can help to reduce the production of histamine, which can cause coughing, and decongestants can help to reduce nasal congestion and make it easier to cough up mucus. Corticosteroids can be used to reduce inflammation in the nasal passages and sinuses.

2.   Nasal irrigation: Nasal irrigation is a technique that involves flushing the nasal passages with a saline solution to help clear mucus and reduce inflammation. It can be helpful in managing allergies and sinusitis, as it can help to reduce nasal congestion and coughing.

3.   Avoiding triggers: Identifying and

avoiding triggers that can cause coughing, such as pollen, dust, and pet dander, is an important aspect of managing allergies and sinusitis.

4.  Steam therapy: Steam therapy can help to reduce coughing by loosening mucus and reducing inflammation in the nasal passages and sinuses. It can be done by taking a hot shower or using a humidifier.

5.  Allergen immunotherapy: Allergen immunotherapy, also known as allergy shots, can help to reduce coughing by reducing the body's sensitivity to allergens. It involves receiving injections of allergens over a period of time to help the body become less sensitive to them.

6.  Surgery: Surgery may be considered for some individuals with chronic sinusitis, such as functional endoscopic sinus surgery (FESS) to open up blocked sinuses and improve breathing.

7.  Saline nasal sprays: Saline nasal sprays can help to reduce coughing by moisturizing the nasal passages and reducing inflammation. They can be used to relieve symptoms of allergies and sinusitis.

8.  Acupuncture: Acupuncture is a form of traditional Chinese medicine that involves the insertion of thin needles into specific points on the body. It can help to reduce coughing by reducing inflammation and promoting relaxation.

9.  Hydration: Staying hydrated is important

for managing allergies and sinusitis, as it can help to thin mucus and make it easier to cough up. Drinking plenty of water, clear fluids, and warm beverages can help to keep the nasal passages and sinuses hydrated.

10.   Practice good hygiene: Wash your hands frequently to reduce the risk of infection and cover your mouth and nose when coughing or sneezing.

11.   Educating oneself: Educating oneself about allergies and sinusitis, their symptoms and triggers, and treatment options can help to better manage these conditions and reduce coughing.

### *Coughing due to Allergies:*

Allergies are a common cause of coughing, and can lead to a range of symptoms that can be both uncomfortable and disruptive to daily life. If you are experiencing a persistent cough that is not relieved by other remedies, it is important to understand the connection between coughing and allergies and to seek the appropriate medical care. Coughing in allergies occurs when your body tries to remove an irritant from your respiratory tract. This can be caused by a wide range of allergens, including pet dander, mold, dust mites, and pollen. When you come into contact with an allergen, your body produces histamine, a substance that causes inflammation and irritation in the airways. This can lead to a range of symptoms, including coughing, wheezing, and shortness of breath.

Diagnosis of allergies typically begins with a thorough medical history and physical examination. If your doctor suspects that you have allergies, you may need to undergo additional diagnostic tests, such as skin prick testing or a blood test, to determine the specific allergens that are causing your symptoms. Once a diagnosis is confirmed, your doctor will work with you to develop a management plan that includes treatment and follow-up care.

Treatment for allergies can vary, depending on the severity of your symptoms and the underlying cause. Options may include allergen avoidance, medications, such as antihistamines or decongestants, or immunotherapy. In some cases, a combination of treatments may be necessary to achieve the best results.

There are several things you can do to help manage your symptoms and prevent complications, and promote a full recovery:

- Reduce your exposure to allergens: To the extent possible, try to reduce your exposure to allergens that are causing your symptoms. This may include keeping your home clean and dust-free, using air purifiers, or avoiding pets if you are allergic to animal dander.

- Practice good respiratory hygiene: Cover your mouth and nose when coughing or sneezing and wash your hands frequently to prevent the spread of germs.

- Stay hydrated: Drinking plenty of fluids can help to thin mucus and prevent dehydration.

- Monitor your symptoms: Keep track of your symptoms, including the frequency and severity of your coughing, and share this information with your doctor.

### *Coughing due to Gastroesophageal Reflux Disease (GERD):*

Gastroesophageal Reflux Disease (GERD) is a condition in which acid from the stomach flows back into the esophagus, causing a range of symptoms, including heartburn, regurgitation, and coughing. GERD can be a particularly challenging condition for individuals who experience coughing as a result of the condition. GERD is caused by a number of factors, including a weak lower esophageal sphincter, which allows stomach acid to flow back into the esophagus. Other factors that contribute to GERD include hiatal hernias, obesity, and certain medications, such as aspirin and other non-steroidal anti-inflammatory drugs (NSAIDs).

Diagnosis of GERD typically involves a thorough medical history and physical examination, as well as diagnostic tests, such as an upper endoscopy, which allows your doctor to visualize the inside of your esophagus and stomach.

Treatment for GERD typically involves managing the underlying cause of the condition and relieving symptoms.

1. Medications: Gastroesophageal reflux

disease (GERD) is managed with medications such as proton pump inhibitors (PPIs) and H2 receptor blockers, which help to reduce acid production in the stomach and prevent acid reflux. These medications can help to reduce symptoms of GERD, such as coughing, heartburn, and chest pain.

2. Lifestyle changes: Making lifestyle changes, such as avoiding triggers, such as spicy, fatty, acidic foods, alcohol, and coffee, and not eating late at night, can help to reduce symptoms of GERD and coughing.

3. Maintaining a healthy weight: Maintaining a healthy weight can help to reduce symptoms of GERD and coughing, as excess weight can put pressure on the stomach and cause acid reflux.

4. Elevating the head of the bed: Raising the head of the bed (about 6-8 inches) by placing blocks or a foam wedge under the mattress can help to reduce coughing and other symptoms of GERD by preventing acid from flowing back into the esophagus.

5. Quit smoking: Quitting smoking can help to reduce symptoms of GERD and coughing, as smoking can relax the lower esophageal sphincter and increase acid production in the stomach.

6. Wear comfortable clothing: Wearing comfortable clothing, such as loose-fitting clothing, can help to reduce symptoms of

GERD and coughing, as tight clothing can put pressure on the stomach and cause acid reflux.

7.  Chewing gum: Chewing gum can help to reduce symptoms of GERD and coughing, as it can stimulate the production of saliva, which can neutralize acid in the esophagus.

8.  Avoiding lying down after eating: Avoiding lying down after eating can help to reduce symptoms of GERD and coughing, as lying down can cause acid to flow back into the esophagus. Eat smaller, more frequent meals: Eating smaller, more frequent meals can help to reduce the risk of reflux and minimize symptoms.

9.  Stress management: Stress can cause the muscles in the esophagus to relax, which can lead to acid reflux. Managing stress through techniques such as deep breathing, meditation, and yoga can help to reduce symptoms of GERD and coughing.

10. Alginates: Alginates are a type of medication that forms a barrier on top of the stomach contents, preventing acid from flowing back into the esophagus and throat, which can reduce symptoms of GERD and coughing.

11. Surgical options: Surgery, such as Nissen fundoplication, can be considered for some individuals with GERD who do not respond to other treatment options. This

procedure can help to reduce acid reflux and coughing by strengthening the lower esophageal sphincter.

12. Monitoring symptoms: Regularly monitoring symptoms, such as coughing, heartburn, and chest pain, is an important aspect of managing GERD. Keeping a symptom diary can help individuals and healthcare providers identify triggers and track the effectiveness of treatment.

### Coughing due to Bronchiectasis

Bronchiectasis is a medical condition characterized by the widening and damage of the airways in the lungs, leading to persistent coughing and difficulty breathing. Coughing is a common symptom of bronchiectasis and it often persists for a long period of time. The cough is usually productive, meaning that it produces mucus, and it may be accompanied by other symptoms, such as wheezing, chest pain, and shortness of breath. As the disease progresses, the coughing may become more persistent and debilitating. The coughing in bronchiectasis is a result of the damaged airways becoming infected with bacteria. This infection can lead to the production of mucus, which can then become trapped in the airways and cause coughing. The coughing helps to clear the airways and to prevent the build-up of mucus, but it also increases the risk of transmitting the disease to others.

Treatment for bronchiectasis typically involves a combination of antibiotics and other medications to manage infections and to reduce inflammation in the airways. In some cases, surgery may be necessary to remove damaged sections of the airways.

Treatment options for bronchiectasis include:

- Medications:
- Bronchodilators, such as albuterol, which help to relax and open up the airways, making it easier to breathe.
- Steroid inhalers, such as fluticasone, which reduce inflammation in the airways.
- Mucolytics, such as acetylcysteine, which help to break down and expel mucus from the lungs.
- Antibiotics, to treat and prevent infections.
- Anti-inflammatory medications such as azithromycin, to reduce inflammation and prevent exacerbations.
- Oxygen therapy: This therapy is used to increase the oxygen level in the blood for people with severe bronchiectasis.
- Pulmonary rehabilitation: A program that includes exercise training, education, and counseling to help improve breathing, muscle strength, and overall fitness.
- Surgery: In some cases, surgery may be considered, such as brachioplasty or lung transplantation, but it's usually reserved for people with severe and progressive disease.

### Coughing due to Pneumonia:

Pneumonia is a serious respiratory condition that occurs when the air sacs in the lungs become inflamed and fill with fluid or pus. This can cause symptoms such as cough, fever, chest pain, and shortness of breath. Coughing is a common symptom of pneumonia, and can range from a mild, occasional cough to a persistent, hacking cough that produces mucus. Understanding the connection between coughing and pneumonia can help you better manage your symptoms and prevent complications. Pneumonia can be caused by a variety of factors, including bacteria, viruses, fungi, and other microorganisms. The condition can be community-acquired, meaning it is contracted outside of a hospital setting, or hospital-acquired, meaning it is contracted while in a hospital or other healthcare facility. Pneumonia can also be classified as mild, moderate, or severe, depending on the severity of the symptoms.

Diagnosis of pneumonia is typically based on a combination of medical history, physical examination, and diagnostic tests, such as chest X-rays, blood tests, and sputum cultures. Once a diagnosis of pneumonia is made, your doctor will work with you to develop a management plan that includes medications, oxygen therapy, and regular follow-up visits.

Treatment for pneumonia typically involves antibiotics, which can help to kill the microorganisms causing the infection. Other medications may also be prescribed to manage symptoms, such as cough suppressants or expectorants to help reduce coughing and improve mucus production. In some cases, oxygen therapy may be necessary to help improve breathing and manage symptoms.

In addition to these measures, there are several things you can do to help manage your symptoms and prevent complications, and promote a full recovery:

- Take your medications as prescribed: Follow your doctor's instructions for taking your medications, including the correct dosing and frequency.

- Get plenty of rest: Pneumonia can be a draining condition, and it is important to get plenty of rest to help your body recover.

- Practice good respiratory hygiene: Cover your mouth and nose when coughing or sneezing and wash your hands frequently to prevent the spread of germs.

- Stay hydrated: Drinking plenty of fluids can help to thin mucus and prevent dehydration.

- Monitor your symptoms: Keep track of your symptoms, including the frequency and severity of your coughing, and share this information with your doctor.

*Coughing due to Chronic Obstructive Pulmonary Disease (COPD):*

Chronic Obstructive Pulmonary Disease (COPD) is a progressive lung disease that makes it difficult to breathe. COPD is characterized by a persistent cough, wheezing, and a feeling of tightness in the chest. In addition to these symptoms, individuals with COPD may also experience shortness of breath, fatigue, and difficulty exercising. COPD is caused by several factors, including long-term exposure to irritants, such as tobacco smoke, air pollution, and workplace dust and chemicals. In addition, other risk factors for COPD include a history of frequent respiratory infections, a family history of lung disease, and a personal history of smoking.

Diagnosis of COPD typically involves a thorough medical history and physical examination, as well as diagnostic tests, such as spirometry, which measures lung function, and imaging studies, such as a chest X-ray or CT scan.

Treatment for COPD typically involves managing the underlying cause of the condition, relieving symptoms, and preventing complications.

- Medications: Both asthma and COPD are managed with medications such as bronchodilators and steroids to help open up the airways and reduce inflammation, making it easier to cough up mucus. Inhaled corticosteroids are commonly used to control asthma symptoms and prevent exacerbations. Long-acting bronchodilators are also commonly used in combination with inhaled corticosteroids to manage COPD.
- Inhalers: Inhalers are devices that deliver

medication directly to the lungs, and are commonly used to manage asthma and COPD. They come in different forms, such as metered-dose inhalers, dry powder inhalers, and nebulizers.

- Avoiding triggers: Identifying and avoiding triggers that can cause coughing, such as smoke, dust, pollen, and chemical fumes, is an important aspect of managing asthma and COPD.

- Pulmonary rehabilitation: Pulmonary rehabilitation is a program that includes exercise, education, and support for individuals with lung disease. It can help to improve lung function and reduce coughing in people with asthma and COPD.

- Oxygen therapy: Oxygen therapy is a medical procedure that involves the delivery of oxygen to the lungs, which can help to reduce coughing and improve breathing in people with COPD.

- Surgery: Surgery may be considered for some individuals with COPD, such as lung volume reduction surgery or lung transplant, to remove damaged lung tissue and improve lung function.

- Flu and Pneumonia vaccination: People with asthma and COPD are at a higher risk of complications from flu and pneumonia, getting vaccinated can help prevent exacerbation and reduce coughing.

- Air purifiers: Using air purifiers can help to reduce exposure to triggers that can cause coughing, such as dust, mold, and pet dander, and can help to improve overall air quality in the home.

- Monitoring symptoms: Regularly monitoring symptoms, such as coughing, shortness of breath, and chest tightness, is an important aspect of managing asthma and COPD. Keeping a symptom diary can help individuals and healthcare providers identify triggers and track the effectiveness of treatment.
- Support groups: Joining a support group for individuals with asthma and COPD can provide emotional and social support, as well as access to information and resources that can help to manage coughing associated with these conditions.
- Educating oneself: Educating oneself about the condition and its management is important for managing asthma and COPD. Understanding the disease, its triggers, and treatment options can help individuals to better manage their condition and reduce coughing.
- Action plan: Having an action plan in place, developed in collaboration with a healthcare provider, is important for managing asthma and COPD. The plan should include information on how to recognize symptoms, how to respond to exacerbations, and when to seek medical attention. The plan could include:

    - Quit smoking: Quitting smoking is the single most effective way to slow the progression of COPD and prevent complications.

- Avoid exposure to irritants: Avoiding exposure to irritants, such as tobacco smoke, air pollution, and workplace dust and chemicals, can help to minimize symptoms and prevent the progression of COPD.

- Exercise regularly: Participating in regular physical activity, such as walking or cycling, can help to improve lung function, reduce symptoms, and promote overall health.

- Maintain a healthy weight: Maintaining a healthy weight can help to reduce the strain on your lungs, prevent complications, and improve overall health.

### Coughing due to Sarcoidosis

Sarcoidosis is a chronic medical condition characterized by the formation of small clusters of inflammatory cells, called granulomas, in various organs and tissues throughout the body, including the lungs. Coughing is a common symptom of sarcoidosis and it may persist for a long period of time. The cough is usually dry and persistent, and it may produce little or no mucus. In some cases, the cough may be accompanied by other symptoms, such as shortness of breath, fatigue, and weight loss. As the disease progresses, the coughing may become more persistent and debilitating.

The coughing in sarcoidosis is a result of the granulomas causing irritation and inflammation in the airways. This irritation and inflammation can lead to the production of mucus, which can then become trapped in the airways and cause coughing. The coughing helps to clear the airways and to prevent the build-up of mucus, but it also increases the risk of transmitting the disease to others.

Treatment for sarcoidosis is typically focused on managing symptoms and slowing the progression of the disease. This may include medications, such as corticosteroids, to reduce inflammation, and oxygen therapy to help improve breathing. In some cases, other medications may be necessary to manage symptoms and to improve quality of life. Treatment options for sarcoidosis include:

Medications:

•        Corticosteroids, such as prednisone, which can help to reduce inflammation and slow down the progression of the disease.

•        Immunosuppressants, such as methotrexate and azathioprine, which can help to suppress the immune system and reduce inflammation.

•        Biologic medications, such as infliximab, adalimumab and etanercept, which can help to reduce inflammation and prevent exacerbations.

Oxygen therapy: This therapy is used to increase the oxygen level in the blood for people with severe sarcoidosis.

Pulmonary rehabilitation: A program that includes

exercise training, education, and counseling to help improve breathing, muscle strength, and overall fitness.

Surgery: In some cases, surgery may be considered, such as lung volume reduction surgery or lung transplantation, but it's usually reserved for people with severe and progressive disease.

Lifestyle Changes:
•        Avoid environmental irritants: Polluted air, dust, chemical fumes, and other irritants can worsen sarcoidosis symptoms.
•        Proper nutrition: A balanced diet can help to maintain weight and muscle strength.
•        Flu and pneumonia vaccinations: To prevent infections that can worsen sarcoidosis symptoms.

In addition to medical treatment, individuals with sarcoidosis may also benefit from supportive care. This may include lifestyle changes, such as quitting smoking, eating a healthy diet, and getting plenty of rest. Supportive care may also involve emotional and psychological support, such as talking to a therapist or joining a support group. It's important to note that sarcoidosis is a chronic, progressive disease, and treatment will depend on the stage of the disease, the symptoms, and the overall health of the patient. Consult with your healthcare provider to develop a personalized treatment plan that is tailored to your individual needs.

### Coughing due to Lung Tuberculosis (TB)

Lung tuberculosis, also known as TB, is a bacterial infection that primarily affects the lungs. Coughing is a common symptom of lung TB, and it can be both a source of discomfort and a means of transmitting the disease to others. Coughing is a common symptom of lung TB, and it often persists for several weeks or months. The cough is usually dry and persistent, and it may produce little or no mucus. In some cases, the cough may be accompanied by other symptoms, such as chest pain, shortness of breath, fatigue, and weight loss. If left untreated, the cough in lung TB can become increasingly persistent and debilitating.

Coughing in lung TB is a result of the bacterial infection causing inflammation in the airways. This inflammation can lead to the production of mucus, which can then become trapped in the airways and cause coughing. The coughing helps to clear the airways and to prevent the build-up of mucus. However, it also increases the risk of transmitting the disease to others.

Treatment for lung TB typically involves a combination of antibiotics and other medications. The goal of treatment is to eliminate the bacteria and to prevent the spread of the disease to others. Antibiotics are the mainstay of treatment for lung TB, and they must be taken as prescribed by a doctor. Other medications, such as cough suppressants, may be prescribed to relieve the coughing and to reduce the risk of transmitting the disease to others. The most common treatment for TB is a combination of several antibiotics, which are taken for a period of six to nine months. The specific medications that are used will depend on the specific strain of bacteria that is causing the infection and your individual circumstances. Some common medications that may be used to treat TB include:

- Isoniazid (INH)
- Rifampin
- Ethambutol
- Pyrazinamide

It is important to take the full course of antibiotics as prescribed by your doctor, even if you start to feel better, to ensure that the infection is fully treated. It is also important to seek medical attention if your symptoms worsen or do not improve.

In addition to medical treatment, individuals with lung TB may also benefit from supportive care. This may include lifestyle changes, such as quitting smoking, eating a healthy diet, and getting plenty of rest. Supportive care may also involve emotional and psychological support, such as talking to a therapist or joining a support group.

### Coughing due to Pulmonary Fibrosis

Pulmonary fibrosis is a lung condition that causes scarring in the lungs, which leads to difficulty breathing and persistent coughing. Pulmonary fibrosis is a chronic medical condition characterized by the formation of fibrous tissue in the lungs. This fibrous tissue can cause the lung tissue to become thick and stiff, leading to difficulty breathing and a persistent cough. Coughing is a common symptom of pulmonary fibrosis and it often persists for a long period of time. The cough is usually dry and persistent, and it may produce little or no mucus. In some cases, the cough may be accompanied by other symptoms, such as shortness of breath, fatigue, and weight loss. As the disease progresses, the coughing may become more persistent and debilitating.

The coughing in pulmonary fibrosis is a result of the fibrous tissue causing irritation and inflammation in the airways. This irritation and inflammation can lead to the production of mucus, which can then become trapped in the airways and cause coughing. The coughing helps to clear the airways and to prevent the build-up of mucus, but it also increases the risk of transmitting the disease to others.

Treatment options for pulmonary fibrosis include:

Medications:

Corticosteroids, such as prednisone, which can help to reduce inflammation and slow down the progression of the disease.

Immunosuppressants, such as azathioprine and mycophenolate mofetil, which can help to suppress the immune system and reduce inflammation.

Antifibrotic medications, such as pirfenidone and nintedanib, which can help to slow down the progression of fibrosis.

Oxygen therapy: This therapy is used to increase the oxygen level in the blood for people with severe pulmonary fibrosis. Oxygen therapy can be administered through a nasal cannula or a face mask. It can be used at home or on the go, and it can help to improve quality of life and reduce the risk of hospitalization.

Pulmonary rehabilitation: A program that includes exercise training, education, and counseling to help improve breathing, muscle strength, and overall fitness.

Surgery: In some cases, surgery may be considered, such as lung volume reduction surgery or lung transplantation, but it's usually reserved for people with severe and progressive disease.

Lifestyle Changes:

Avoid environmental irritants: Polluted air, dust, chemical fumes, and other irritants can worsen pulmonary fibrosis symptoms.

Proper nutrition: A balanced diet can help to maintain weight and muscle strength.

Flu and pneumonia vaccinations: To prevent infections that can worsen pulmonary fibrosis symptoms.

Supportive care. This may include quitting smoking, eating a healthy diet, and getting plenty of rest. Supportive care may also involve emotional and psychological support, such as talking to a therapist or joining a support group.

It's important to note that pulmonary fibrosis is a chronic, progressive disease, and treatment will depend on the stage of the disease, the symptoms, and the overall health of the patient. Consult with your healthcare provider to develop a personalized treatment plan that is tailored to your individual needs.

### Coughing due to Lung Cancer

Lung cancer is a serious and often life-threatening condition that occurs when abnormal cells in the lung tissue grow and multiply uncontrollably. There are two main types of lung cancer, small cell lung cancer and non-small cell lung cancer, and both can cause a wide range of symptoms, including coughing. Understanding the connection between coughing and lung cancer can help you better manage your symptoms and prevent complications.

Coughing can be a sign of lung cancer for a variety of reasons. In some cases, the coughing may be caused by the presence of a tumor that is obstructing the airways. This can lead to a persistent, hacking cough that produces mucus. In other cases, the coughing may be caused by irritation or inflammation of the airways, which can occur as a result of the cancer spreading to other parts of the body.

Diagnosis of lung cancer typically begins with a thorough medical history and physical examination. If your doctor suspects that you have lung cancer, you may need to undergo additional diagnostic tests, such as a chest X-ray, CT scan, or biopsy. If a diagnosis of lung cancer is confirmed, your doctor will work with you to develop a management plan that includes treatment and follow-up care.

Treatment for lung cancer can vary, depending on the stage and type of the cancer, as well as your overall health and medical history. Options may include surgery, radiation therapy, chemotherapy, or a combination of these treatments. In some cases, medications may also be prescribed to manage symptoms, such as cough suppressants or expectorants to help reduce coughing and improve mucus production.

In addition to these measures, there are several things you can do to help manage your symptoms and prevent complications:

- Take your medications as prescribed: Follow your doctor's instructions for taking your medications, including the correct dosing and frequency.

- Get plenty of rest: Lung cancer can be a draining condition, and it is important to get plenty of rest to help your body recover.

- Practice good respiratory hygiene: Cover your mouth and nose when coughing or sneezing and wash your hands frequently to prevent the spread of germs.

- Stay hydrated: Drinking plenty of fluids can help to thin mucus and prevent dehydration.

- Monitor your symptoms: Keep track of your symptoms, including the frequency and severity of your coughing, and share this information with your doctor.

### Coughing due to Congestive Heart Failure (CHF)

Coughing can be a sign of a number of underlying medical conditions, including cardiac issues. When coughing is related to a cardiac issue, it is often referred to as a "cardiac cough." One of the most common causes of a cardiac cough is congestive heart failure (CHF), a condition in which the heart is unable to pump enough blood to meet the body's needs. This can result in fluid buildup in the lungs, leading to a persistent, hacking cough.

Other cardiac issues that can cause a cough include heart valve disease, such as aortic stenosis, in which a narrowed valve makes it difficult for blood to flow from the heart to the rest of the body, and pulmonary hypertension, a condition in which the blood pressure in the pulmonary artery is elevated.

Diagnosis of a cardiac cough typically involves a thorough medical history and physical examination, as well as diagnostic tests, such as an electrocardiogram (ECG), echocardiogram, and chest X-ray.

Treatment for a cardiac cough depends on the underlying cause and may involve medications, such as diuretics to remove fluid from the lungs, or heart valve surgery to repair or replace damaged heart valves.

There are several things you can do to help manage your symptoms and prevent complications:

- Take medications as prescribed: Taking medications, such as diuretics, as prescribed can help to relieve symptoms, prevent complications, and improve overall health.

- Exercise regularly: Participating in regular physical activity, such as walking or cycling, can help to improve cardiovascular function, reduce symptoms, and promote overall health.

- Maintain a healthy diet: Eating a healthy, balanced diet can help to control weight, reduce blood pressure, and improve cardiovascular function.

- Manage stress: Finding healthy ways to manage stress, such as through exercise, meditation, or therapy, can help to reduce symptoms, improve overall health, and prevent complications.

### *Coughing due to Respiratory Syncytial Virus (RSV)*

Respiratory syncytial virus (RSV) is a highly contagious virus that causes respiratory infections in individuals of all ages, including infants, children, and adults. Coughing is a common symptom of RSV and it may persist for several days or weeks. The cough is usually dry and persistent, and it may be accompanied by other symptoms, such as wheezing, shortness of breath, and fever. As the disease progresses, the coughing may become more persistent and debilitating, leading to difficulty breathing and increased risk of complications.

The coughing in RSV is a result of the virus causing inflammation and irritation in the airways. This inflammation and irritation can lead to the production of mucus, which can then become trapped in the airways and cause coughing. The coughing helps to clear the airways and to prevent the build-up of mucus, but it also increases the risk of transmitting the disease to others.

Treatment for RSV is typically focused on relieving symptoms and preventing complications. This may include medications, such as antivirals, to help manage symptoms and reduce the duration of the infection, as well as supportive care, such as plenty of rest and fluids, to help the body recover. In some cases, oxygen therapy or hospitalization may be necessary to manage symptoms and to prevent serious complications. Treatment options for RSV include:

Antiviral medications: There is currently no specific antiviral medication that is approved for the treatment of RSV. However, some research has suggested that the use of ribavirin, an antiviral medication, may be effective in certain cases of severe RSV infection.

- Symptomatic treatment:
- Over-the-counter medications, such as acetaminophen or ibuprofen, can help to reduce fever and relieve pain.
- Decongestants, such as pseudoephedrine, can help to relieve nasal congestion.
- Cough suppressants, such as dextromethorphan, can help to reduce coughing.

- Supportive care:
- Drinking fluids to stay hydrated.
- Using a humidifier to moisten the air and help relieve nasal congestion.
- Getting plenty of rest.

- Hospitalization:
- In some cases, hospitalization may be necessary for people who are having difficulty breathing, or for those who are at high risk for complications.

- Care at home:

- For most people with RSV, the infection will resolve on its own with proper self-care. This includes getting plenty of rest, drinking fluids to stay hydrated, and using over-the-counter medications to relieve symptoms.

- Prevention:
- Prevention in high-risk individuals: Some people are at higher risk for severe RSV infection, such as premature infants, older adults, and people with underlying medical conditions. For these individuals, preventive measures, such as palivizumab, a monoclonal antibody, may be given during the RSV season to reduce the risk of severe infection.

- Prevention in healthcare settings: To prevent the spread of RSV in healthcare settings, it's important to follow infection control guidelines, such as proper hand hygiene, isolation precautions, and respiratory hygiene.

- Wash your hands frequently to reduce the risk of infection.

- Supportive care: This may include lifestyle changes, such as avoiding close contact with others and practicing good hygiene to prevent the spread of the virus. Supportive care may also involve emotional and psychological support, such as talking to a friend or loved one about your concerns and fears.

- Get vaccinated against RSV, although there is no specific vaccine for RSV.

- Surgery: In rare cases, surgery may be necessary to treat a persistent cough. For example, surgery may be needed to remove a foreign object that is stuck in the airway or to repair damage to the airway.

It's important to note that RSV is a common virus and most people who are infected will recover without any problems. However, some people are at higher risk for severe illness and complications, such as premature infants, older adults, and people with underlying medical conditions. If you or your child has symptoms of RSV, it's important to consult with a healthcare provider to ensure that proper care is given and to monitor the symptoms.

### Coughing due to SARS-CoV-2 Virus (Covid-19)

Coughing is a common symptom of the novel coronavirus disease (COVID-19), caused by the SARS-CoV-2 virus. It is often one of the first symptoms to develop and can range from a mild, occasional cough to a severe, persistent cough that produces mucus or phlegm. The exact mechanism by which the virus causes coughing is not fully understood, but it is believed to be related to the way the virus affects the respiratory system. The virus enters the body through the nose or mouth and attacks the cells that line the airways, causing inflammation and irritation. This can lead to coughing, as well as other respiratory symptoms, such as shortness of breath, wheezing, and chest pain.

In some cases, coughing can be a sign of a more severe form of COVID-19, known as acute respiratory distress syndrome (ARDS). ARDS is a life-threatening condition that can occur when the body's immune system overreacts to the virus and damages the lungs, making it difficult to breathe.

Diagnosis of COVID-19 is typically based on symptoms, as well as a positive result from a molecular diagnostic test, such as a reverse transcription polymerase chain reaction (RT-PCR) test. Treatment for COVID-19 typically involves supportive care, such as rest, hydration, and over-the-counter pain medications, to relieve symptoms.

Treatment for coughing caused by COVID-19 will depend on the severity of the illness. The main goal of treatment is to relieve symptoms and prevent complications. If you have mild symptoms, such as a mild cough, you may be able to manage them at home with self-care measures. Some effective ways to alleviate coughing caused by COVID-19 include:

Hydration: Keeping yourself hydrated by drinking water, clear broths, frozen water or ice chips, clear teas, frozen fruit juices can help to thin mucus and make it easier to cough up. Drinking plenty of fluids to help keep mucus thin and easier to cough up.

Steam therapy: Inhaling steam can help to moisturize your airways and make it easier to cough up mucus. You can use a humidifier, take a hot shower, or boil water and breathe in the steam. Using steam therapy could add moisture to the air and help soothe a dry throat.

Saltwater gargle: Mixing a teaspoon of salt with a cup of warm water and gargling can help soothe a sore throat and reduce the urge to cough.

Nasal irrigation: Using a saline nasal spray can help to flush out mucus and reduce congestion in the nasal passages, which can make it easier to breathe and cough.

Inhaling essential oils: Essential oils such as eucalyptus, peppermint and thyme can help to alleviate coughing.

Over the counter medication such as cough syrups, paracetamol and ibuprofen.

Resting as much as possible. Avoiding smoking or second-hand smoking. Practicing good hygiene such as washing hands, covering your mouth and nose when you cough or sneeze, and avoiding close contact with sick people.

It's important to note that these self-care measures are not a substitute for medical care and should be used in conjunction with the guidance of a healthcare professional. If your symptoms worsen or do not improve after a few days, it's important to seek medical attention.

If you have moderate to severe symptoms, you may need to be hospitalized. In this case, your healthcare provider may give you oxygen therapy, mechanical ventilation, and other treatments. It's important to follow the guidance of your healthcare provider, and if you have any concern, seek medical attention.

Antiviral medications are drugs that can help to reduce the severity and duration of a viral infection by inhibiting the virus's ability to replicate.

If you have a cough due to Covid-19, your healthcare provider may recommend antiviral medications as part of your treatment plan. Currently, the following antiviral medications are authorized for the treatment of Covid-19:

1. Remdesivir: This is an intravenous medication that is used to treat severe cases of Covid-19.

2. Favipiravir: This is an oral medication that is used to treat mild to moderate cases of Covid-19.

3. Dexamethasone: This is a corticosteroid that is used to reduce inflammation in the respiratory tract. It may be used to treat severe cases of Covid-19.

It is important to note that these medications may not be appropriate for everyone and can have potential side effects. It is important to follow the dosing instructions for any medications that are prescribed to you and to seek medical attention if your symptoms worsen or do not improve.

It's important to remember that preventing COVID-19 is still the best way to avoid getting sick, so it's important to follow the guidance of public health officials and take measures to protect yourself and others, such as wearing a mask, practicing physical distancing, and washing your hands regularly. It's also important to note that if you have COVID-19, you should follow the guidance of public health officials and stay in isolation to avoid spreading the virus to others.

# CHAPTER 20

## *Support Groups and Online Resources for Coughing*

C oughing is a common condition that affects millions of people worldwide. While coughing is usually a symptom of an underlying condition, it can also be a standalone issue that can cause discomfort and distress. To manage coughing and its symptoms, it is essential to seek the help of a healthcare provider. A doctor can diagnose the underlying cause of your coughing and recommend the appropriate treatment. However, many people with coughing also benefit from joining a support group or accessing online resources for coughing. These resources can provide information, support, and coping strategies for those who are dealing with coughing.

Support groups for coughing can be found both in-person and online. In-person support groups provide an opportunity for people with coughing to connect with others who are going through similar experiences. These groups can offer a supportive environment where people can share their stories, ask questions, and offer advice. In-person support groups may be led by a healthcare provider, a trained facilitator, or a peer.

Online support groups for coughing are also available. These groups are typically hosted on websites or social media platforms and are open to anyone who is dealing with coughing. Online support groups provide a convenient and accessible option for those who are unable to attend in-person support groups. These groups also offer a large and diverse community of people who are dealing with coughing, making it easier to find someone who is facing similar challenges.

- Support groups and online resources can be an important source of support and information for people who are coping with coughing. They can provide a sense of community and a place to share experiences and learn from others who are going through similar struggles.
- Support groups can be found in various settings such as hospitals, community centers, and online platforms. They provide a space for individuals to connect with others who are going through similar experiences and to receive emotional support, information, and guidance.
- Online resources can be a helpful tool for managing coughing and finding relief. Websites, blogs, and forums can provide information on treatments, coping strategies, and research on coughing.
- Many support groups and online resources for coughing are dedicated to specific conditions such as asthma, bronchitis, and chronic obstructive pulmonary disease (COPD) that can cause coughing.
- Support groups and online resources can provide a sense of community and belonging, which can be especially important for people who are isolated or dealing with a chronic condition.

- Online resources can also provide access to the latest research and information on coughing and its treatments, which can be helpful for individuals who are looking for a more comprehensive understanding of their condition.

- Support groups and online resources can also provide a space for individuals to ask questions, share personal experiences and learn from others who have gone through similar experiences.

- Support groups and online resources can be a helpful tool for individuals who are looking for additional support and information beyond what they receive from their healthcare providers.

- Support groups are a great way to connect with others who are coping with coughing and to find support, encouragement, and information. These groups can provide a sense of community and belonging and can be a valuable source of information and resources.

- Support groups can be found in person, such as at hospitals, clinics, and community centers, or online through social media platforms and websites.

- Online support groups can provide a convenient and accessible way to connect with others who are coping with coughing, regardless of location.

- Support groups can be specific to a particular condition, such as asthma or bronchitis, or more general, such as a chronic cough support group.

- Joining a support group can also help to reduce feelings of isolation and provide a sense of empowerment, as individuals can share their experiences and learn from others.

- Online resources such as websites, forums, and blogs can provide a wealth of information on coughing and its management. These resources can provide information on causes, symptoms, treatments, and coping strategies.
- Online resources can also provide information on the latest research and developments in coughing, as well as updates on new treatments and medications.
- Online resources can also provide information on support groups, both online and in-person, and can help connect individuals with others who are coping with coughing.
- Online resources can also provide information on lifestyle changes, such as diet and exercise, that can help to manage coughing.
- Online resources can also provide information on alternative therapies.

In addition to support groups, there are also many online resources available for those who are dealing with coughing. Websites, forums, and social media groups provide information on coughing and its causes, treatments, and coping strategies. These resources also offer a platform for people to ask questions and receive answers from healthcare providers and other knowledgeable individuals.

Some online resources for coughing include:

- The American Lung Association: This organization provides information on coughing and its causes, as well as tips for managing symptoms and seeking treatment.

- Mayo Clinic: This website provides comprehensive information on coughing and its causes, as well as information on treatment options and lifestyle changes that can help manage symptoms.

- National Heart, Lung, and Blood Institute: This organization provides information on coughing and its causes, as well as information on treatment options and lifestyle changes that can help manage symptoms.

- WebMD: This website provides information on coughing and its causes, as well as information on treatment options and lifestyle changes that can help manage symptoms.

- American Academy of Allergy, Asthma, & Immunology: This organization provides information on coughing and its causes, as well as information on treatment options and lifestyle changes that can help manage symptoms.

The management of persistent coughs depends on the underlying cause(s) and the severity of the cough. Here are some general principles of cough management:

- Relief of symptoms: The primary goal of cough management is to relieve symptoms and improve quality of life. This may involve the use of over-the-counter (OTC) or prescription medications, such as cough suppressants, expectorants, decongestants, and bronchodilators, as well as natural remedies and home remedies.

- Prevention of complications: Persistent coughs can lead to complications, such as muscle strain, headaches, rib fractures, and even hernias. Therefore, it is important to take measures to prevent these complications, such as using proper coughing techniques and avoiding heavy lifting. If chest pain, shortness of breath and even dyspnea occurred after frequent severe coughing, the rupture of bullae caused pneumothorax. The lung tissue could be compressed, and the situation was critical. The closed chest drainage could been performed by a thoracic surgeon immediately.

- Treatment of underlying causes: To resolve a persistent cough, it is essential to treat the underlying cause(s). This may involve the use of antibiotics for respiratory infections, allergy medications for allergies, and inhalers for asthma and COPD.

○ Lifestyle modifications: Making lifestyle changes, such as quitting smoking, avoiding exposure to irritants, and managing stress, can help prevent persistent coughs and improve respiratory health.

In conclusion, coughing is a common condition that can cause discomfort and distress. Support groups and online resources can provide information, support, and coping strategies for those who are dealing with coughing. Whether you choose to attend an in-person support group or access online resources, it is important to seek the help of a healthcare provider to manage your symptoms and receive a proper diagnosis.

## CHAPTER 21

# *Emotional and Psychological Support for Coughing*

Coughing is a common medical condition that can be caused by various factors, including respiratory infections, allergies, irritants, and certain medical conditions. Although coughing can help clear the airways, it can also lead to physical discomfort, stress, and anxiety. Emotional support is a crucial aspect of managing coughing. Individuals who suffer from frequent coughing episodes may feel frustrated, embarrassed, and helpless. They may feel like their cough is impacting their daily life and causing them to miss out on social activities. To provide emotional support, it is important to be a good listener, to be understanding, and to offer reassurance and encouragement. Showing empathy and concern for their struggles can help to reduce their stress and anxiety.

Psychological support is also an important part of managing coughing. Individuals may experience a range of negative emotions, such as anxiety, fear, and depression. These emotions can lead to a decrease in self-esteem and overall well-being.

Frustration: Coughing can be an annoying and exhausting symptom, and it can be frustrating when it persists or interferes with daily activities.

Anxiety: A persistent cough can be a sign of an underlying health problem, and this can cause anxiety about the cause of the cough and potential treatment options.

Depression: Coughing can be a physically and emotionally draining symptom, and it can take a toll on a person's overall well-being. In some cases, this can lead to feelings of depression.

To provide psychological support, it is important to educate individuals about the condition and its potential causes. This will help them to understand the condition better and to feel more in control. Additionally, it is important to encourage individuals to seek professional help, such as seeing a doctor or a therapist, if their symptoms are affecting their quality of life. To cope with the emotional and psychological aspects of a cough, it can be helpful to:

Seek support: It can also be helpful to talk to a healthcare provider or mental health professional if you are struggling to cope with the emotional and psychological impact of a cough. Talking to a healthcare provider, a therapist, or a support group can provide emotional support and help you cope with the impact of the cough on your quality of life. They can provide additional support and resources to help you manage these feelings.

Seek treatment: Receiving proper treatment for the underlying cause of the cough can help alleviate symptoms and improve quality of life.

Practice self-care: Taking care of yourself,

including getting enough rest, staying hydrated, and managing stress, can help improve overall health and well-being.

Set realistic goals: It's important to be realistic about what you can and cannot do while you are dealing with a cough. Setting achievable goals and finding ways to adapt to any limitations can help improve your overall sense of control and well-being.

In conclusion, coughing can have a significant impact on an individual's emotional and psychological well-being. By providing emotional and psychological support, as well as practical strategies, individuals who are struggling with coughing can find relief and improve their quality of life. It is important to remember that everyone's experience with coughing is unique and that support should be tailored to each individual's needs. If you or someone you know is struggling with coughing, seek professional help for a comprehensive evaluation and treatment plan.

## CHAPTER 22

## *Conclusion*

## *Finding Lasting Solution for Coughing*

Coughing is a common condition that affects millions of people worldwide. It can be a symptom of an underlying condition or a standalone issue that can cause discomfort and distress. Finding lasting relief from coughing requires a multi-pronged approach that involves seeking the help of a healthcare provider, making lifestyle changes, and seeking support from others.

Try home remedies: Home remedies, such as inhaling steam, using a humidifier, and drinking warm liquids, can help relieve coughing symptoms. It is important to speak to your healthcare provider before trying any home remedies.

Alternative therapies: such as acupuncture, acupressure, yoga and breathing exercises, Ayurvedic medicine, Traditional Chinese medicine, chiropractic care, massage therapy, aromatherapy, and mind-body therapies can provide relief from coughing and address the underlying cause of the coughing.

Use over-the-counter remedies: Over-the-counter remedies, such as cough drops and decongestants, can help relieve coughing symptoms. It is important to follow the instructions on the label and speak to your healthcare provider before using these remedies.

Making changes to your lifestyle can help manage symptoms of coughing. This may include quitting smoking, avoiding exposure to irritants, and managing stress levels. Drinking plenty of water can help keep your mucous membranes moist and reduce the severity of coughing. Aim to drink at least eight glasses of water per day.

Join a support group: Joining a support group can provide a supportive environment where you can connect with others who are dealing with coughing. Support groups can be found both in-person and online and are a great way to find information, support, and coping strategies for those who are dealing with coughing.

Access online resources: There are many online resources available for those who are dealing with coughing. Websites, forums, and social media groups provide information on coughing and its causes, treatments, and coping strategies. These resources also offer a platform for people to ask questions and receive answers from healthcare providers and other knowledgeable individuals. Don't hesitate to reach out to support groups and online resources if you need additional support and information.

Seek the help of a healthcare provider: A doctor can diagnose the underlying cause of your coughing and recommend the appropriate treatment. It is important to seek the help of a healthcare provider as soon as possible to ensure prompt and effective treatment. Although traditional prescription drugs can provide relief from coughing, they may have side effects and may not address the underlying cause of the coughing. It's important to communicate with healthcare providers and practitioners about your specific condition and goals, and to be open to exploring different options for managing coughing. Keep track of your symptoms, triggers, and treatment progress to help identify patterns and make adjustments to your treatment plan as needed.

Lifestyle changes such as quitting smoking, avoiding triggers, staying hydrated, and getting enough rest can also help to alleviate coughing and improve overall respiratory function. Consider trying a combination of different therapies to find the most effective approach for managing coughing. Be consistent with your treatment plan and stick to the recommended schedule, to allow enough time for the therapy to take effect.

It is also important to note that some alternative therapies may interact with other medications or have contraindications, and it's important to communicate with a healthcare provider or qualified practitioner before starting any new treatment. In addition to the tips previously mentioned, it is also important to note that coughing can be a sign of an underlying serious condition such as pneumonia or lung cancer, so it's important to see a healthcare provider if the coughing persists or is accompanied by other symptoms such as chest pain, difficulty breathing, or a persistent high fever.

It is important to remember that a healthy lifestyle is the foundation of a strong immune system. By making healthy choices and taking care of yourself, you can help to support your immune system and reduce your risk of illness.


In conclusion, finding lasting relief from coughing requires a multi-pronged approach that involves seeking the help of a healthcare provider, making lifestyle changes, and seeking support from others. By following these tips and takeaways, you can find relief from coughing and improve your overall quality of life. However, it is important to remember that everyone's experience with coughing is unique and it may take time to find what works best for you.

Printed in Great Britain
by Amazon